Power-Packed Food
for Sports + Adventure

ROCKET
FUEL

MATTHEW KADEY, RD

VELO press

Boulder, Colorado

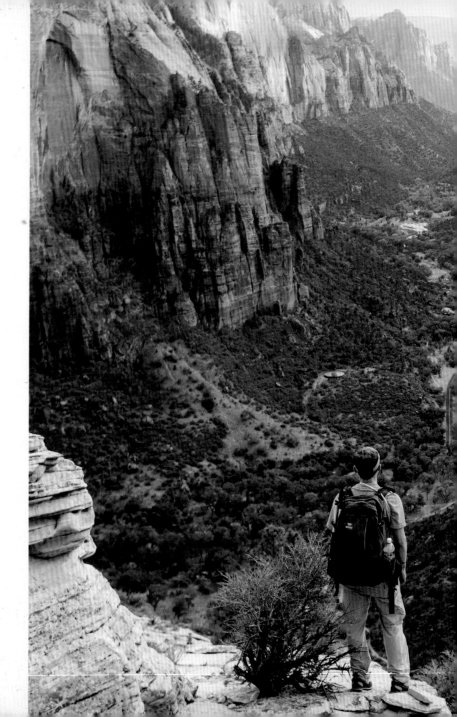

velopress®

3002 Sterling Circle, Suite 100, Boulder, Colorado 80301-2338 USA
(303) 440-0601 · Fax (303) 444-6788
E-mail velopress@competitorgroup.com

Distributed in the United States and Canada by Ingram Publisher Services

Library of Congress Cataloging-in-Publication Data
Names: Kadey, Matt.
Title: Rocket fuel : power-packed food for sports and adventure /
  Matthew Kadey, RD.
Description: Boulder, Colorado : VeloPress, c2016. | Includes bibliographical
  references and index.
Identifiers: LCCN 2015042481 | ISBN 9781937715465 (pbk. : alk. paper) |
  ISBN 9781937716790 (e-book)
Subjects: LCSH: Nutrition. | High-carbohydrate diet. | High-protein diet.
Classification: LCC RA784 .K225 2016 | DDC 613.2—dc23
LC record available at http://lccn.loc.gov/2015042481

For information on purchasing VeloPress books,
please call (800) 811-4210, ext. 2138, or visit www.velopress.com.

This paper meets the requirements of
ANSI/NISO Z39.48-1992 (Permanence of Paper).

Cover design: **Andy Omel**

Art direction and interior design: **Vicki Hopewell**

Cover and recipe photography: **Aaron Colussi**, also pp. ii, iv, 18, 27, 32, 76, 150

Adventure photography: **Michael Clark**, p. 88; **Liam Doran**, pp. 3, 152;
Myke Hermsmeyer, pp. viii, 22, 72, 140, 226; **Matthew Kadey**, pp. 25, 148,
247, 248; **iStock/Lorado**, p. 86; **iStock/Charles Shug**, p. 145; **Thinkstock**,
pp. 29, 75

Food styling by **Eric Leskovar**

16 17 18 / 10 9 8 7 6 5 4 3 2 1

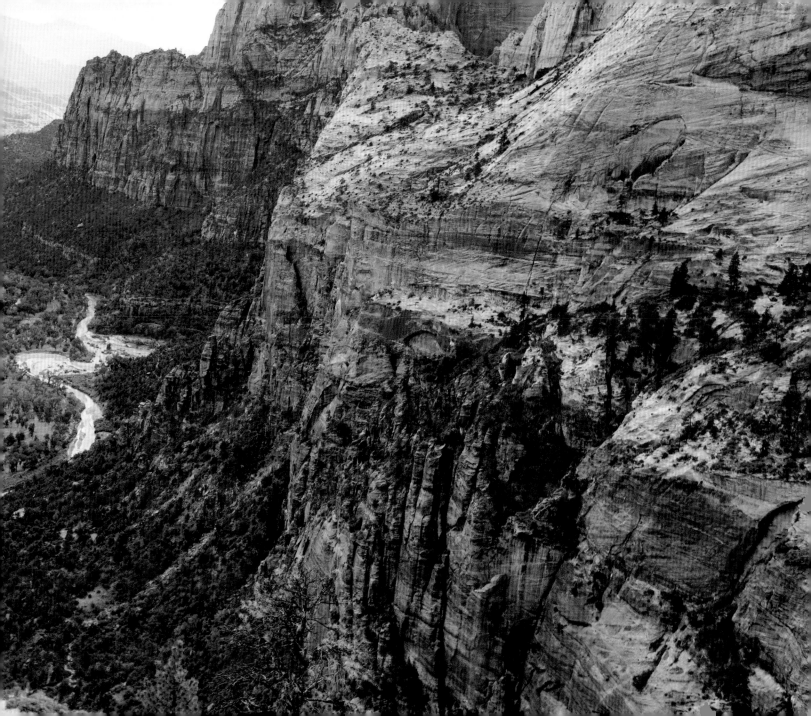

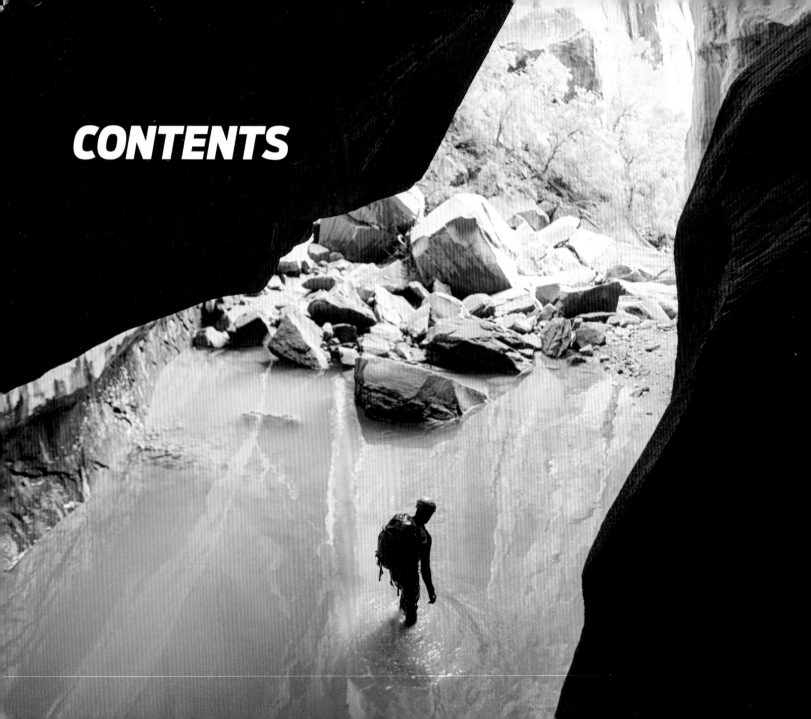

CONTENTS

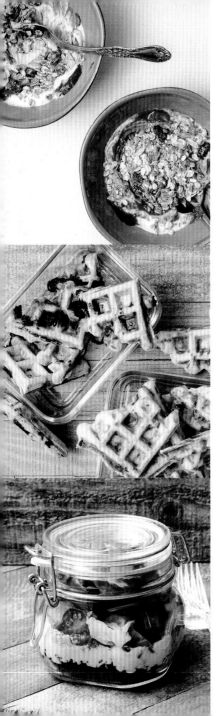

BEFORE

DURING

AFTER

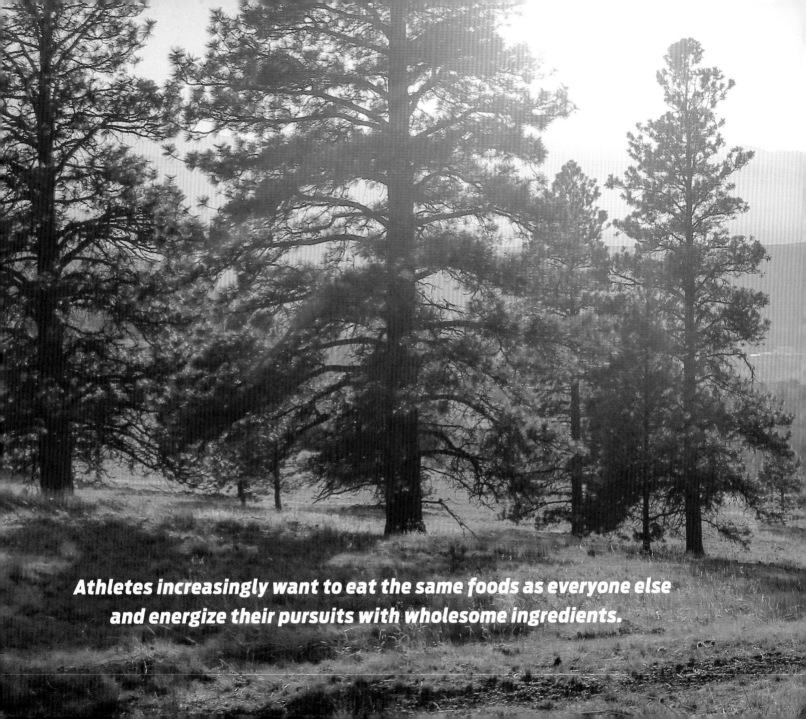

Athletes increasingly want to eat the same foods as everyone else and energize their pursuits with wholesome ingredients.

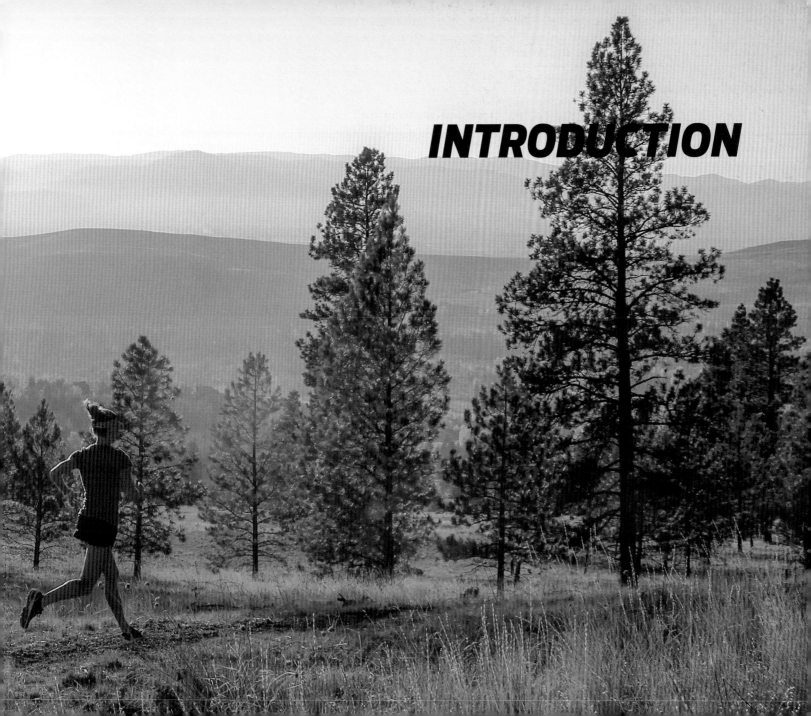

INTRODUCTION

As any seasoned athlete or adventure seeker will attest, what you put in your stomach BEFORE, DURING, and AFTER exercise can mean all the difference between a winning performance and one that won't make any headlines.

To be a champion, you have to eat like one. You don't want to let your hard work on the saddle, in the gym, or on the field go to waste by not fueling properly. If your competition is eating optimally for performance and you're taking nutrition lightly, you shouldn't be surprised when you get left in the dust.

Even though no one food can turn a donkey into a racehorse and produce an instant athlete, consuming the right combination of foods and drinks on a daily basis can go a long way in helping you train harder and longer. In turn, good workouts will make the most of good nutrition practices. So whether you are a frequent Tough Mudder, mountain bike racer, bodybuilder, or mountaineer preparing for your next summit, good nutrition over the long haul is a key aspect of a successful fitness regimen. In other words, think marathon, not sprint, when it comes to sports nutrition and healthy eating.

With that in mind, when you're heading out for a run, ride, paddle, or hike in the great outdoors, it can be tempting to stuff your jersey pockets and backpack full of packaged sports nutrition products that promise to deliver peak performance. Before and after exercise are times you might find yourself swayed by the convenience and touted benefits of those products. And with daily life feeling more time-crunched than ever, why would you bother trading in the portable, ready-to-use packaged bars, gels, and their ilk for homemade fuel? It's a valid question indeed, but when you take a closer look at the pros and cons of either option, it's one that can be answered with resounding support for fuel from your own kitchen.

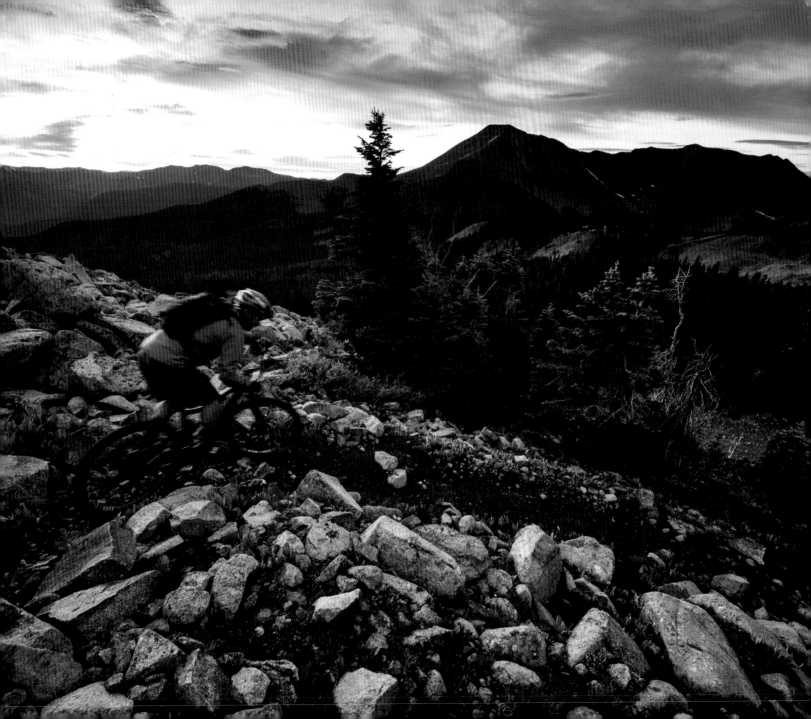

BACK *TO THE* KITCHEN

WHILE THE ORIGINS of the premade, packaged energy-food market can be disputed, few would argue that the release of the malleable, malt-flavored PowerBar in the '80s was a launching pad for what has now become a multibillion-dollar business. Sure, its cardboard-like taste was appetite killing and it would turn harder than carbon when temperatures dipped, but athletes suddenly had a convenient source of energy that they could stash in their gym bags or backpacks and turn to in a flash.

In the years since, the market has been flooded with a dizzying array of engineered products that run the gamut from powders to bars designed to provide athletes of all stripes with specialized fuel. As society as a whole abandoned their kitchens in droves in response to increasing demands on time, these products continued to rise in popularity and even transcended the role of workout fuel to become regular snacks and meals. Professional athletes with sizable sponsorship deals have been all too happy to plug one product or another as a means of achieving athletic greatness. And the rise in popularity of sporting events such as marathons, Gran Fondo road races, and mud runs has only served to fuel the packaged-fuel biz. Heck, you can now even subscribe to delivery services where a box of bars, chews, and sticky gels arrives at your front door monthly—exercise fuel in your hands without moving a muscle.

Despite the size and prevalence of this prepackaged food industry, a powerful movement is now afoot among athletes and adventurers. They are increasingly ignoring the sea of sales pitches and flashy packaging and instead once again turning back to energy food created in their own kitchens to power their active lifestyles. Food blogs, Pinterest, and other social media platforms are being saturated with recipes from pro athletes as well as weekend warriors, all offering up tasty ideas for homemade bars, sports drinks, and copious other sweet and savory performance-fuel options. These athletes are committed to raising the bar, so to speak, on sports nutrition. It's never been a better time to be a fit foodie.

While the day of the prepackaged gel and bar hasn't yet come and gone, and likely won't ever disappear, there is a broad movement in sports nutrition toward once again embracing real food. More people are becoming aware of the potential benefits of ditching some of the store-bought stuff

for made-with-love forms of performance nutrition that keep them naturally fit.

Most important, diet has become the new essential and important arena that athletes are scrutinizing to find competitive gains. No longer is the athletic crowd using their workouts as an excuse to stuff themselves silly on boxed cereal and frozen pizza with too many multisyllabic ingredients. Instead, amateurs and pros alike are applying the same level of intensity and focus to their eating habits as they do to their training and competition. That's because it's now well understood that sound nutrition is a vital element in overall performance.

Keeping this in mind, athletes are becoming cognizant that healthy eating does not just apply to mealtime but also to the fuel they pump into their bodies before, during, and after workouts. This means that people are increasingly asking themselves why athletes are fueling life's adventures with items made from high-fructose corn syrup and mystery flavoring when they could energize their pursuit with more wholesome local honey and real fruit. Kitchen-savvy athletes understand that ingredients such as nuts, fruits, and whole grains used as the backbone for more natural forms of energy also deliver a bounty of nutrients necessary for overall well-being. In short, homemade sports nutrition is simply an extension of the wider pull toward a more nutritious overall diet.

Further, people are increasingly skeptical about the ingredients found in many forms of engineered sports foods. For too long, packaged sports products have benefited from a health halo owing to their association with athletics. But now, athletes who have regularly turned to these items for a fitness boost are scrutinizing ingredient lists—and what they're seeing is not always appetizing. Some of the same ingredients you would find in supermarket foods, like highly processed sugars and preservatives deemed to be "junk food," are also all too common in a number of sports nutrition items. Sure, lab-created sports foods are convenient and popular, but are they actually optimal fuel for an overall healthy body? For many people, it's about having more control over what they put in their bodies and stressing quality over convenience. Sometimes simpler is better.

As much as we'd all like to think we're riding an innovative new wave in this turn to homemade sports foods, the concept of real food as athletic fuel isn't without precedent. The numerous forms of athletics existed well before gels and chews flooded the market, and somehow athletes still were able to cross the finish line. The Olympians of yesteryear who weren't able to quaff Gatorade understood that Mother Nature knows a thing or two about fueling active pursuits. Before sports drinks, bars, and neon goo became race-day staples, athletes tapped the produce, bread, and dairy aisles for a competitive edge. In fact, the engineered sports-food phenomenon is still very much rooted in North American society. In Europe and South America, for example, you won't see the sheer variety of packaged energy foods on offer here. When the athletic crowd on other continents is feeling peckish, they may very well reach for a sandwich rather than a bar. If you need proof that you can go fast without relying solely on PowerBars and their counterparts, just look in the musette bags of Grand Tour riders, which can include tasty treats ranging from rice cakes to panini.

I'm also an ardent believer in real-food fuel, both from my perspective as a dietitian and as a cyclist. I've cycled thousands of miles in dozens of countries without needing to overload my panniers with bars and gels. (OK, I once had to rely on a few too many energy bars in Cuba when I couldn't stomach another lackluster peso pizza.) Instead, whenever I've felt hungry and a little sluggish, I've turned to actual food. Save for the rare occurrence of needing to find a bathroom pronto, it has never let me down or left me feeling weak in the legs and wanting extra energy from engineered sports fuel. When I need a power boost, a mound of refreshing papaya salad and pad Thai in Thailand or a handheld pie in Argentina have historically been more of what I crave in nearly every way compared to a brick of tapioca syrup.

Despite my firm preference for real-food fuel, I'll concede that the use of these prepackaged items is often unavoidable and that there will continue to be a market for them (including yours truly), but let me present what I consider a rock-solid case for powering your active lifestyle more often with do-it-yourself, all-natural fuel from your kitchen instead of the science lab.

IT WORKS

As I'll discuss in more detail later on, there is increasing science to support the use of food you find in bulk bins and produce aisles to bolster endurance and strength to the same degree (if not more!) than the stuff created by the white coats. Case in point: *A Journal of the International Society of Sports Nutrition* study found that raisins were just as effective as carbohydrate-based energy chews at keeping runners' endurance levels up. That's why you'll find these little nuggets of energy in one of my homemade Energy Shots (p. 137). Heck, even a lowbrow bowl of cereal and milk has been found to be great recovery fuel. To learn how to make your own without a trip to a cereal aisle populated by additives and chemical coatings, turn to page 160.

NUTRITION UPGRADE

If you're not taking your nutrition seriously, it's likely much of your competition is. This fact alone can be enough to ensure that they leave you playing catch-up. You can train until your legs fall off, but if you don't have your nutrition on point, your fitness gains during training are going to be subpar and it's likely you'll have a tough race. While eating *real* food like spinach may not give you the superhuman strength of a gravel-voiced sailorman, it's a vital aspect of overall power, speed, and endurance. Sound nutrition is also a key part in preventing the injuries and illnesses that can arise from frequent training. So eating well allows you to train much more efficiently.

I often trumpet that one of the most important benefits of giving your pots and pans a workout by making your own edible energy is that it's another opportunity to take in a wider variety of the vital nutrients that an active body requires to perform its best and yield quicker training results. Feeding

INSIDE THE WRAPPER

When it comes to fueling your activity, it's easy to trust the flashy wrappers and promotional buzz of prepackaged products, especially when they're being endorsed by professional athletes in glitzy advertisements and live-event product placement. Think about those carefully positioned bottles of a certain neon sports drink perched on the table in front of athletes and their coaches during postgame press conferences. The prominence of sports nutrition products encourages athletes to take product claims at face value, but more and more athletes are finally taking a closer look at nutrition labels and ingredient lists. And increasingly what they uncover is pushing many back into the kitchen. Don't just take my word for it when I say there can be a lot of additives and other questionable ingredients in prepackaged sports nutrition products: Start checking out those labels for yourself. While there are now, thankfully, an increasing number of whole-food-based fuel options on the market, for the most part you'll still see a pattern: Not only do DIY options often have fewer ingredients, they also lack any that sound completely foreign. Just to illustrate the argument, here's a side-by-side comparison of ingredients in a prepackaged energy bar and a real-food energy option.

Energy Bar, Chocolate

INGREDIENTS

cane invert syrup
maltodextrin
fructose
dextrose
oat bran
soy protein isolate
alkalized cocoa
brown rice flour
high oleic canola oil
vegetable glycerin
calcium phosphate
salt
chocolate
potassium phosphate
sugar
natural flavor
ascorbic acid
partially defatted peanut flour
nonfat milk
ground almonds
ferrous fumerate
pyridoxine hydrochloride
thiamin hydrochloride
riboflavin

Enduro Balls

INGREDIENTS

pitted dates
rolled oats
raw almonds
raw sunflower seeds
raw pumpkin seeds
hemp seeds
ground flaxseed
cocoa powder
salt
honey
almond butter
fresh mint
vanilla extract
chocolate chips

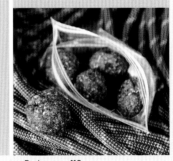

Recipe on p. 110

a body in training is no mean feat, so any opportunity to sneak in more nutrient-dense items such as fruits, veggies, seeds, and whole grains into pre-, during-, and post-workout noshes is surely welcomed.

KEEPING IT REAL

Flip over a packaged sports nutrition product and you'll likely wish you majored in food chemistry. Although items on the market increasingly rely on healthy ingredients that even your grandma would recognize, the norm is still to pack them full of a minefield of mystery items, including food colorings, emulsifiers, "natural flavors," fractionated oils (what?), and artificial sweeteners. I don't know about you, but soy protein nuggets and carnauba wax are not something I have in my pantry or necessarily want to put in my body on a regular basis. Funny how these products can still be labeled "natural." So consider committing to making your own pre-, during-, and post-workout goodies an important step toward mindful and cleaner eating.

TROUBLEMAKERS

For better or worse, an increasing number of athletes are steering clear of certain items such as lactose and gluten. In certain cases, this is a must in response to conditions such as lactose intolerance or celiac disease. Crafting your own fuel affords you better control over sidestepping possible food allergens or ingredients that simply don't fit into the dietary lifestyle you have embraced.

IN GOOD TASTE

Relying heavily on packaged energy-food products can lead to a serious case of palate fatigue. After all, there are only so many cloyingly sweet gels and cat food–like meat bars you can stomach before you want to tap out. Also, the same tastes and textures seem to be pumped out again and again, which can get old quick. Really, another peanut butter and chocolate bar? An underappreciated benefit of homemade fuel is that it can promote better fueling by making you actually want to eat the stuff—and leave your workouts seeming a little more gourmet. Appetite suppression is a big concern among athletes such as Tour de France riders and ultrarunners if they eat the same thing too often. Anyone who racks up the miles knows this firsthand. If I have only brought along packaged gels or bars on a long ride, I'm often underfueling toward the end because the thought of inhaling another raspberry-flavored maltodextrin product is truly unappetizing. And I don't know about you, but I always want to curl up and take a nap instead of hopping on the saddle after eating a bar with yogurt coating that doesn't actually contain yogurt. To extend the shelf life of packaged bars, the moisture is sucked out, which leaves your workout food tasting like lumber. That's why real-food goodies are especially helpful when you are out for the long haul. So consider the recipes populating this book as a means to boosting performance and creating yum in the process. They provide fuel that is as appetizing as it is functional.

VARIETY IS THE SPICE OF LIFE

When you make your own performance fuel, you can have fun experimenting with all sorts of exciting and innovative ingredient to create flavors and textures that will motivate you to trade time sitting in front of a computer for time working up a sweat. That's why I spent countless hours in the kitchen creating these recipes that not only provide useful calories but also push the boundaries of what athletes are accustomed to eating when on the move or in need of recovery sustenance. After all, who says a little prosciutto only belongs on a charcuterie board?

You'll also recognize that fueling your active lifestyle can be so much more than smoothies and bars. Although those recipes are here too, everything from crepes to protein-packed pudding can offer your active body a dynamic duo of great taste and performance benefits.

SAVE CASH

Walk into any bike, running, or outdoor-gear shop and you'll inevitably be greeted by displays of so-called sports nutrition products promising to boost your game. However, their convenience comes with a price tag. Although the occasional use won't break the bank, when you consider that each gel can set you back a couple bucks and some bars ring in at a hefty $4, relying solely on store-bought packaged energy foods can put a serious dent in your gear or race budget. Making your own fitness fuel can leave you more wiggle room for race entry fees or that bucket list bike trip to the Alps. With that said, it's still a good idea to think about quality and not just price when it comes to the ingredients you use. It's easier to pay a little more for sustainable seafood, local honey, fair-trade chocolate, and organic milk if you know that they're a better choice for the planet and your active body.

EAT BETTER OVERALL

A strange thing happens when people decide to take the time to craft their own performance fuel. All of the

FUELING CHEAT SHEET

Here's a quick, at-a-glance guide to what you should consider as you think about food in relation to your workouts.

BEFORE

FUELING

2–3 hours before: Low-glycemic meal with 50–60% carbs, 20–30% protein, 15–30% fat

30–60 min. before: Low- to moderate-glycemic snack low in fiber, moderate fat and protein, 150–300 calories (less calories for light workouts)

Endurance workout: + calories and carbs

Resistance/strength training: + protein

HYDRATION

Add 1–2 cups of fluid to pre-workout routine for morning workouts or an especially hot or sweaty session.

Maintain hydration during the day with calorie-free drinks like water and tea.

TIPS

Focus on whole foods for added nutrients.

Audition fuel during training. Don't try something new before a big race.

DURING*

FUELING

Prioritize carbs: 30–90 g/hour of a workout.

Moderate amounts of fat and protein during prolonged activity are OK.

Resistance training: Some protein can reduce muscle damage.

HYDRATION

Drink 400–1,000 mg/hour.

Replace electrolytes with sodium, at least 300 mg/hour.

TIPS

Try a variety of flavors from real foods to stimulate appetite.

Fuel and hydrate at regular intervals instead of all at once.

The hotter the temperature, the more calories and liquids you need.

AFTER

FUELING

0–60 min. after: 1.25–1.5 g of carbs for each kg body weight

High-intensity endurance exercise: + carbs, moderate protein, less fat; roughly 4-to-1 carb-to-protein ratio

Resistance training: + protein; roughly 2-to-1 carb-to-protein ratio

HYDRATION

Drink water, smoothies, and other fluids.

Get more sodium after sweaty workout.

TIPS

Real food works just as well as packaged alternatives.

Prepare options ahead of time for easier, quicker recovery fueling.

* See page 79 to determine if you need to fuel during your workout.

sudden, they start to get excited about cooking again and increasingly trade in trips to the drive-thru for old-fashioned home cooking. Preparing a batch of ride cookies or post-workout muffins can propel you to look for other ways to infuse your diet with optimal fuel, namely homemade, nutrient-dense breakfasts, lunches, and dinners. Think of it as improved nutrition by osmosis. No longer will you call a bowl of sugary boxed cereal breakfast or settle for a frozen packaged burrito come the dinner bell. It's about taking the time to once again discover the perks of preparing your own food.

As with exercise fuel, by making your own meals you'll have a much better idea of what you are putting in your body, and as long as you cook with quality ingredients such as whole grains, healthy protein, fruits, and vegetables, this will contribute to overall performance and health. The advantage of consuming mostly snacks and meals prepared in your own kitchen was played out in a recent University of Illinois study. It determined that despite their better reputation, meals at higher-end restaurants can actually deliver greater amounts of undesirables such as sodium and cholesterol than do meals from fast-food joints. Regardless of where people ate out, the researchers also found that subjects ended up eating more nutritionally lackluster calories than if they consumed food they prepared with their own two hands.

TASTE THE REWARD

Having an arsenal of go-to fuel recipes can have the positive side effect of encouraging you to exercise with greater frequency. After all, enjoying delicious fuel only really works if you also keep active. I will happily work up a sweat if I can take a bite out of some Salted Quinoa Almond Fudge Cups (p. 225) afterward or bring along a bagful of Sushi Rolls (p. 134).

/////

Rocket Fuel has a clear purpose: to offer up nutritious, tasty, and often simple recipes to fuel your body in the best way possible and help you thrive in your athletic pursuits. In my mind, that means food you make yourself for sustained energy and improved nutrition instead of relying on the fleeting pick-me-ups from manufacturers that often stress quantity over quality. My goal here is to help you discover how amazing it can be to get in the kitchen and pump out an assortment of homemade fuel in as many exciting flavor combinations as possible so you can reach your fitness goals and even surpass them. It's true that on-the-go fuel from the kitchen largely has its roots in the cycling world, but by no means are these recipes geared only toward the Lycra community. A broad spectrum of athletes can benefit from the kitchen creations found here. Whether you plan to tackle some fierce white water, scale a rock face, pump serious iron, shred some powder, prepare for a grueling romp in the mud, or endure a day of bushwhacking, *Rocket Fuel* recipes give you the nutritional building blocks needed to rise to the challenge and perform at your best. In other words, you can fuel your workouts *your* way.

ROCKET FUEL BASICS

YOU'LL FIND A BOUNTY of recipes in this book that are formulated specifically to help you prepare for, sustain, and recover from training and races. Here's how to make them work for you.

CLOCKWORK

The recipes that follow are grouped into three main sections: Before, During, and After. They are designed to meet the needs of pro athletes, the lunch-hour fitness crowd, and weekend warriors alike during these specific times. So, for instance, a post-training recipe such as Pumpkin Pie Yogurt Bowl with Super Seed Sprinkle (p. 163) will have the higher levels of the protein needed to encourage muscle recovery, whereas the During section is full of fuel such as Coconut Rice Cakes (p. 106) that provide plenty of carbs to power your activity of choice. Many recipes, including Chocolate Milk (p. 168) and the Watermelon Slushy (p. 67), are distilled from the latest sports-nutrition science suggesting that they can provide a specific benefit at a specific time for those who like to work up a sweat on a regular basis and who want to go that extra mile.

DIET GUIDE

Within each recipe, you'll find the following letters that let you quickly recognize if a recipe written as is or with some easy tweaking (see the Game Changers) can fit into a particular dietary restriction or if it can be made ahead and preserved for future needs.

D **DAIRY-FREE**

Recipe contains no dairy, such as milk or yogurt, or can be made dairy-free with certain ingredient adjustments. This can include swapping out cow milk for a nondairy alternative such as almond milk. There are now more dairy-free options than ever for items such as butter and cheese.

F **FREEZER-FRIENDLY**

Recipe or elements of the recipe can be frozen if placed in an airtight container, allowing leftovers to be used down the road. These recipes offer athletes the option of making a big batch of fuel without the worry that it will rot in their fridge. They're also a great option for weekend warriors who may want to make a recipe and use it to fuel an active outing on more than one weekend.

G **GLUTEN-FREE**

Recipe contains no gluten-containing ingredients or can be modified to be gluten-free by using alternatives such as an all-purpose gluten-free flour blend instead of wheat flour.

P **PALEO-FRIENDLY**

Recipe adheres to the dietary principals of Paleo eating or can be adjusted to be Paleo. This means no grains, legumes, or refined sugars; however, some Paleo diets allow for dairy, and a recipe with the **P** symbol may include this food group.

V **VEGETARIAN OR VEGAN-FRIENDLY**

Recipe contains no meat (vegetarian) or no meat, dairy, eggs, or honey (vegan), or can be modified to meet one or both of these eating preferences.

By no means is the recipe timing written in stone. Several can be moved around to suit your gastronomic desires. While Cherry Mojito Popsicles (p. 214) aren't likely something you're going to take along on the trail, I'm definitely not opposed to enjoying a Crepe Roll (p. 130) as a pre-workout nibble or a Strawberry Cheesecake Wrap (p. 133) as part of my recovery nutrition.

SWITCH HITS

In many of the recipes, you'll see a section called Game Changers. It provides suggestions for recipe alterations that can be made based on what you have in your pantry, preferred tastes, or any required dietary restrictions. My goal was to make each recipe as accessible as possible to a wide audience, and if you can't find or don't like a certain ingredient, there may be a good replacement. Use these recipes as a launching pad to creating your own edible energy by using your kitchen as a laboratory for experimentation.

In some cases, these recipe alterations also offer an opportunity to adjust a recipe to up the health ante. So while the Brownie Bites (p. 125) call for all-purpose flour for easier digestion when pushing the pace, you can easily swap in a whole-grain flour such as spelt or whole wheat pastry flour to turn them into a healthier snack option.

TOOLS OF THE TRADE

You certainly don't need a fully pimped-out professional kitchen to make your own fuel, but these items can help get the job done with ease.

Blender. Like chocolate, not all blenders are created equal. When it comes to this kitchen workhorse, you'll often get what you pay for. A blender with serious horsepower such as Vitamix, Breville, Ninja, or Blendtec can make quick work of fruits, vegetables, nuts, and frozen items such as bananas when in need of a smoothie fix. Beyond post-workout drinks, a blender with notable wattage can be used to make homemade nut butters, dips, spreads, cocktails, and desserts. I've used my Vitamix several times a day for a number of years, and it's still going strong. When it comes to blenders on the market, there is more competition than ever, so shop around for one that suits your culinary and budgetary needs.

Food processor. Most athletes who enjoy spending some time in the kitchen crafting their own workout fuel come to realize that a food processor is a must-have tool, despite being a bit of a space hog. It's ideal for pulverizing items such as dried fruit, fresh vegetables, and nuts for recipes like energy bars where a blender does not work very well due to the lack of liquid. Many food processors come with attachments for slicing and shredding that can make quick work of vegetables for salads and other needs. My preferred model is the 12-cup Cuisinart, but there are other reliable brands on the market. Weight can be a good indication of the power of the motor.

Digital scale. For more precision when following recipes where ingredients such as dry pasta, potatoes, and chocolate are provided by weight, it's a good idea to stock your kitchen with a digital kitchen scale. The tool is also handy if you're watching your portions of stuff like cheese when trying to maintain a race weight. There are plenty of options on the market at budget-friendly prices.

Cast-iron skillet. The gym isn't the only place where I like to lift some iron. When it comes to making Inside-Out Pancakes (p. 101) and Crepe Rolls (p. 130) to fuel my rides, I always rely on my cast-iron skillet. It's inexpensive, sturdy, nonstick when seasoned right, and can easily go from stove top to oven, also making

it a great option for frittatas, corn bread, and roasted chicken. And unlike your running shoes, with proper care a cast-iron skillet only gets better with age. Most kitchen supply stores carry several options, but you might be able to grab one at a yard sale or from your grandma's attic.

Muffin tins. A trusty muffin tin is a great way to make items in a portable, pre-portioned format. Mini-muffin trays that have 12, 20, or 24 molds (holding about 2 tablespoons of batter each) per tray are well suited for making bite-sized workout treats. Muffin trays with standard-sized cups come with either 6 or 12 molds that hold about a half cup of batter each. I most often call on this size for use in post-workout recipes.

Food-grade silicone muffin trays are my go-to choice for a few reasons. First, they are virtually nonstick, so you won't have to face a sticky situation after cooking. I also appreciate that they are flexible, which makes unmolding items such as Smoothie Cups (p. 170) a simple undertaking. Being able to turn the cups inside out also makes washing them a breeze. What's more, silicone muffin trays are freezer, microwave, and dishwasher safe. You can find silicone muffin trays at most kitchen supply shops.

THE NEW POWER FOODS

It's called fuel for a reason. Just like gas for a car, proper nourishment gives your body the energy it needs to crank out the miles. You certainly don't have to spend the big bucks on obscure Amazonian berries to meet your dietary needs, and my goal for this book was not to construct a bunch of recipes full of hard-to-find so-called superfoods, but it's a good idea to stock your kitchen with these less-than-mainstream nutritional overachievers to give your active body a bounty of nutrients. Find them at health food stores, online, or in an increasing number of larger supermarkets.

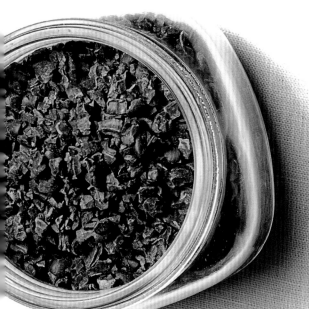

CACAO NIBS

Made by simply smashing up the whole cacao beans used to produce chocolate bars and hot chocolate, this raw form of chocolate is a crunchy way to infuse your diet with plenty of antioxidants, minerals, and dietary fiber. Add them to a bowl of oatmeal, yogurt, or ice cream.

HEMP SEEDS

Also called hemp hearts, these seeds taste like the love child of pine nuts and sunflower seeds. Their impressive nutritional résumé includes healthy amounts of protein, omega fatty acids, and magnesium. Use them in DIY energy bars and balls, and sprinkle generous amounts on cereal, yogurt, and soups.

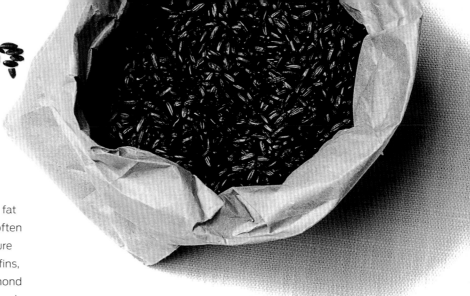

ALMOND FLOUR

This grain-free, gluten-free flour contains several nutritional highlights, including higher levels of protein, vitamin E, and healthy monounsaturated fat than typical wheat or other grain-based flours. I often use it to add a nutty essence and wonderful texture to recipes. For recipes such as pancakes and muffins, try replacing about a quarter of the flour with almond flour. You can also use it to make flourless items such as Flourless Protein Banana Muffins (p. 209).

CHIA SEEDS

Chia has experienced a renaissance as a functional food thanks to its high levels of fiber, healthy fats, antioxidants, and minerals. You can sprinkle the mild-flavored seeds on oatmeal, salads, and yogurt or take advantage of their ability to absorb huge amounts of water for use in healthier puddings and fruit spreads.

DRIED TART CHERRIES

Although it is very difficult to find fresh tart cherries, the dried version is readily available and ready to help you recover with research-proven antioxidants. Dried tart cherries also contain some melatonin to help you snag some recovery z's. On top of their use in several of the recipes in this book, work them into pancake and muffin batter, salads, and even pasta dishes.

BLACK RICE

This heirloom variety of rice from Asia that also goes by the name Forbidden Rice has a great chewy texture and slightly sweet taste. Research shows that it possesses a payload of the same health-hiking anthocyanin antioxidants found in dark berries such as blueberries. This makes up-and-coming black rice an excellent way to infuse your diet with whole-grain carbohydrate energy.

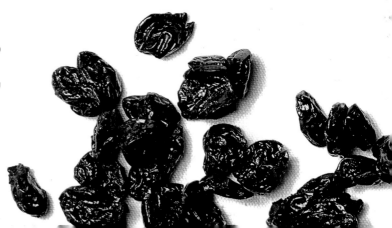

If you are going to go the metal route, I recommend purchasing a muffin tray made with heavy-gauge steel such as aluminized or stainless steel, which allows for even heating and produces perfectly browned baked items. When you pick up the pan, you want it to feel solid and have some weight to it. Also, look for a tray with large, wide handles, making it easier to slide into and out of the oven.

Silicone baking mat. A reusable silicone baking mat such as Silpat eliminates the need for greasing your baking sheets or lining them with single-use foil or parchment paper. They're great for making everything from roasted vegetables to ride cookies to Granola Yogurt Bark (p. 223).

Zester. Somehow cooking existed before the zester, a low-key tool that proves that awesome things come in small packages. The tiny razor-edge holes make hundreds of fine cuts on foods such as citrus peel, which I use in many of the recipes in this book to add a punch of bright flavor minus the engineered flavorings added to many store-bought fuel options. Beyond grating citrus, I use it for Parmesan cheese, garlic, ginger, fresh turmeric root, and even chocolate. Think of it as a way to add micro-hits of flavor.

Wraps. Fuel items in this book such as Millet Cherry Bars (p. 102) and Waffle Bites (p. 97) need to be wrapped tightly for transport when you are on the go. There are a few options for getting the job done. Parchment foil, which is essentially parchment-lined aluminum foil, is durable and holds its shape very well. The parchment side also provides a nonstick surface, which is great when you are wrapping up sticky items. A standard heavyweight aluminum foil can also get the job done. For portable fuel, I also encourage trying a more eco-conscious reusable option such as Abeego, which is made with earth-friendly and anti-bacterial hemp, organic cotton, and beeswax. I'd advise against using flimsy plastic wrap, which can make for a messy mid-ride nosh.

Jars. If you spend any time on Instagram or Pinterest, you know that ye olde food canning jars are back in fashion. Forward-thinking cooks are layering all sorts of food into jars for near-instant meal satisfaction. For harried athletes, having pre- and post-training snacks and meals such as Raspberry Chia Pudding (p. 40) or Instant Miso Noodle Soup (p. 196) stuffed into jars at the ready can offer the opportunity for rapid fueling or refueling when you need it most.

Cooler. A cooler comes in handy for transporting temperature-sensitive items so you can have nourishment ready for you when you return to your car or the trailhead. There are numerous brands on the market in a variety of sizes to meet your needs. Generally, you should expect to pay a little more for one that will keep your food cooler for longer.

Thermos. A solidly built thermos such as Hydro Flask can keep hot foods hot and cold foods cold for several hours, which is great for transporting chilly or sultry fuel options such as smoothies or porridge on the road.

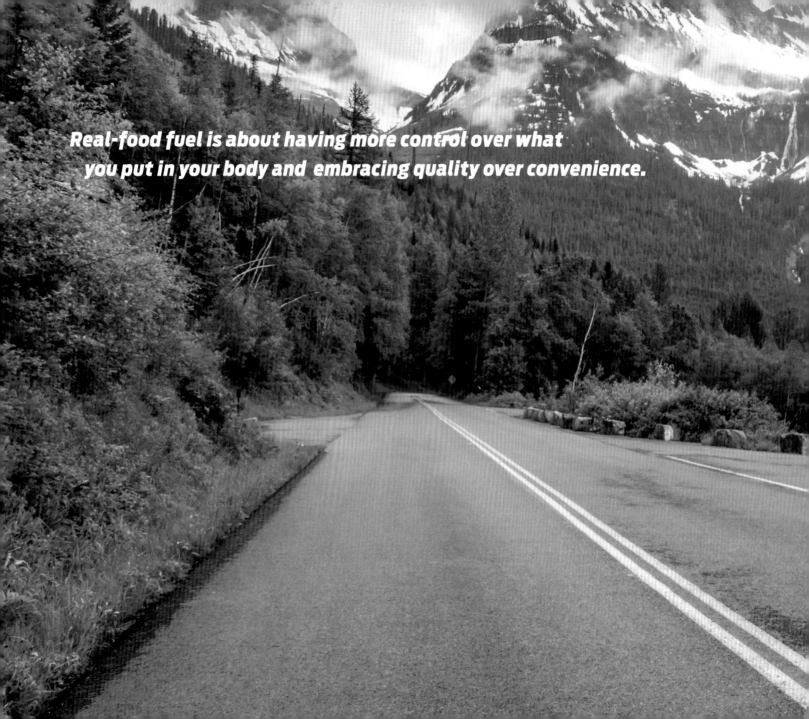

Real-food fuel is about having more control over what you put in your body and embracing quality over convenience.

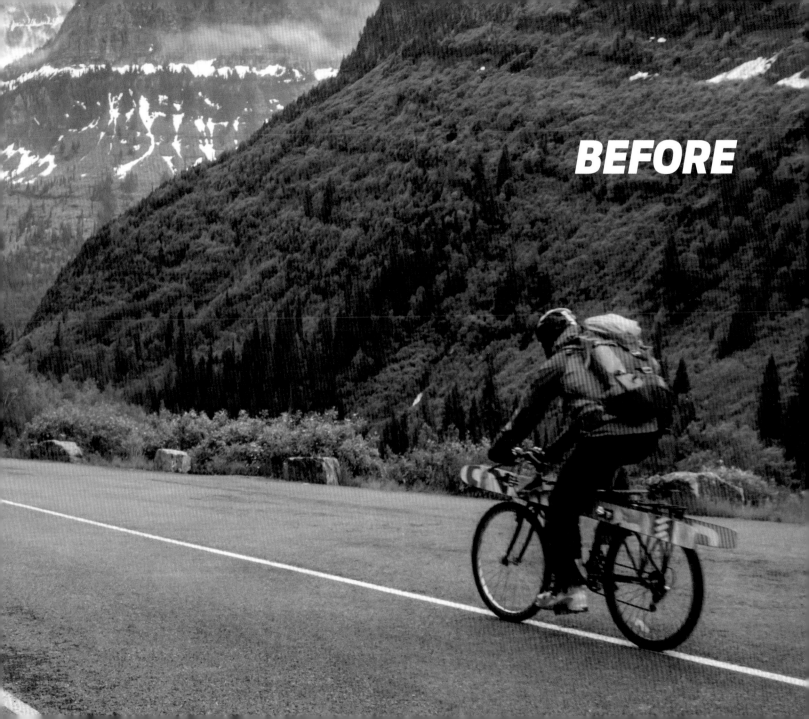

BEFORE

START *YOUR* ENGINE

AS A SPORTS DIETITIAN, I frequently field questions from athletes who want to know what to eat to get a good boost of energy to go strong from the get-go.

If you're heading out for an ambitious ride or making your way to the gym for a lively workout after a day at the office, it's a good idea to take a preemptive strike and fuel your body. For breakout success, you should take your pre-workout fuel just as seriously as your post-workout nutrition. After all, there are few people who can podium or bag a summit on an empty stomach or one that is full of empty calories.

Pre-exercise nutrition serves a number of important functions that can mean the difference between a workout that is bragworthy and one that falls flat. For starters, making the right fuel choice before working out can give you the energy burst you need to jump-start your exercise regimen. By helping keep your blood sugar levels steady, a pre-workout nibble plays a big role in allowing you to maintain an intense pace during the initial stages of your training, race, or CrossFit WOD so you don't prematurely toss in the towel. That's because this sugar floating around in your body enhances the availability of fuel to your active muscles. Drops in blood sugar caused by skipping your pre-workout fueling or making poor food choices might result in light-headedness and fatigue, and ultimately cause you to fade early.

Eating something before you crush some treadmill sprints or kick up the dirt can also serve to top off your glycogen stores. This is particularly important for hard training that is going to take a big bite out of this essential energy reserve or if you are taking part in morning exercise, where the overnight fast has tapped into your glycogen stores and blood sugar is likely on the low end.

Without optimal fuel, your workouts are bound to be less productive or intense than they could be because you'll suffer from premature fatigue—an outcome that not only brings about reduced training gains but also results in fewer calories being burned during exercise, which can hinder weight-loss efforts in people who are trying to slim down. If a pre-exercise snack helps you go harder to burn more calories overall, consider it an investment in building a lean, mean body.

A nibble before hitting the water, field, or pavement can also go a long way in squashing performance-sapping hunger pangs during exercise, which are an indication that your body could have

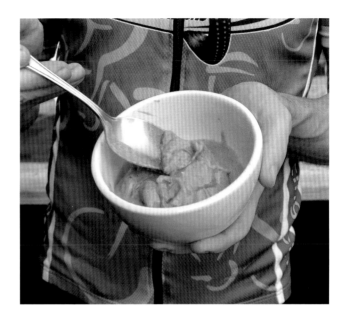

used more fuel. Being preoccupied with a growling stomach means you'll have less mental power available to focus on your workout and the technique needed to perform at your best. I know for certain that I'm less likely to pick the best lines on our local mountain bike trails if I have visions of doughnuts dancing in my head because I bolted out the door before eating enough chow.

Healthy pre-workout foods also help athletes meet their overall calorie and nutrient needs. Items such as bananas, dried fruit, and nuts contain an arsenal of vitamins, minerals, and antioxidants that are essential for an active body to perform at its best. So consider your pre-workout fuel as being functional for both short-term performance and long-term health.

Often overlooked is the fact that pre-exercise fueling, particularly with carbohydrates, can keep athletes healthy by helping to lessen the drop in immunity that the body can experience in response to intense workouts. The immune suppression that occurs with high-volume training or following intense bouts of exercise can sideline you with illnesses such as upper respiratory tract infections. Science shows that carbohydrate fueling before and during vigorous exercise is one potential way to help keep the doctor at bay.

With all this said, you don't want to eat the wrong thing before you head out for a workout. Here are some general guidelines to follow.

AUDITION YOUR FUEL

Undeniably, pre-workout feeding is a highly personal endeavor. Through trial and error during training (read: not just before a big race), you have to determine how much you can eat and what food combinations work for you for the given situation. For example, I can eat a fair amount of food before a workout and find that I perform better on the bike with a fairly full belly. Others with more sensitive guts need to wait an hour or more between eating and working out or they risk feeling too sluggish or suffering a serious case of digestive woes as the pace picks up. In the end, you need to pay attention to what works for you during training and eat that or something very similar before stepping up to the starting line. You know your stomach best.

TIMING IS EVERYTHING

Most athletes perform their best when they consume a larger meal that contains carbs, protein, and healthy fats 2 to 3 hours before a workout and then a smaller snack consisting of 150 to 300 calories 30 to 60 minutes before showtime. This allows sufficient time to digest the calories of a large meal and also gives you a hit of pre-workout nutrition for a little boost without leaving you feeling heavy and lethargic. But by "large" I don't mean a stuff-yourself-silly buffet-style meal. You want your meal to be almost totally digested before you grab a lighter snack and head to the gym. Again, the timing of your pre-workout meals needs to be individualized to what works for you based on experience. Trial and error is the surest way to pinpoint your happy zone.

GO SLOW

Much of the energy in your pre-workout meal should come from carbohydrates, but you may want to save your homemade energy shots and sports drinks for during exercise. Science shows that consuming a lower-glycemic-index meal or snack before working out—which raises your blood sugar at a slower clip—can bring about notable performance benefits. When you consume a high-glycemic item such as a chew, a flood of insulin is released to remove the sugar from your blood. This can cause a sudden drop in blood sugar that may leave you feeling bonky early on during exercise. Nobody wants to feel drained when the workout has just begun.

It also turns out that chomping on lower-glycemic foods can encourage more fat-burning during exercise, which spares your glycogen stores for when you need to call upon them to crank up the pace and improve endurance capacity. Elevated fat-burning can also benefit those who are using exercise as one means of slimming down. Turning to complex carbohydrates such as sweet potatoes and even including a little bit of protein or fat in your pre-workout snack will lower the glycemic index of your fuel, resulting in a gradual release of carbs into your bloodstream that makes for more consistent energy levels during your workout so you can keep your motor humming.

DON'T ROUGH IT

From reducing the risk of heart disease to making it less likely you'll develop a set of love handles, a high-fiber diet is vital to athletes' overall well-being. But it's best not to spoon up a lentil salad shortly before working out. Too much fiber in your pre-exercise nosh can greatly slow down digestion, leading to potential digestive issues such as bloating, which is not exactly conducive to a stellar performance. The last thing you want is to feel weighed down when you're trying to nail a Strava segment.

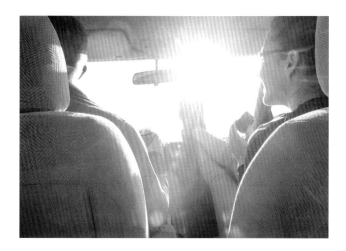

FOR THE LOVE OF CARBS

Rocket Fuel definitely doesn't shy away from embracing carbohydrates for optimal performance. But carb haters have long blamed the macronutrient for everything from brain fog to low energy levels to developing a Buddha belly. Well, two recent studies deservedly show carbs some love and help cut through the amazing amount of noise surrounding their consumption.

Researchers at the National Institute of Diabetes and Digestive and Kidney Diseases recruited 19 overweight individuals and split them into two groups. In an around-the-clock laboratory setting to prevent dietary cheating, one group was fed a low-carb diet for two weeks while the other was provided a low-fat diet. Both groups received the same number of calories, 30 percent fewer than they were accustomed to. The groups then switched diets after a couple weeks of rest from the study. It turns out the average weight loss was about the same, roughly a pound of fat (4 pounds total) over two weeks, no matter which diet was followed. The study's authors concluded that the total calories consumed likely plays a bigger role in achieving and maintaining a healthy body weight than whether you cut down on a certain macronutrient such as carbohydrates or fat. So the upshot is that you don't need to ditch your beloved oatmeal or toast if you want to keep lean as long as you pay attention to how many overall calories—and the quality of those calories—you are taking in.

And it turns out that smart athletes do fuel up on carbohydrates and don't necessarily have to settle for cauliflower-crust pizza. A study published in *The Quarterly Review of Biology* gleaned information from archaeological, anthropological, genetic, physiological, and anatomical data to show that increased carbohydrate consumption, particularly in the form of cooked starch like that found in pasta and potatoes, was the vital dietary change for the evolution of the modern big-brained human. It's believed that additional carbs in the form of more easily digested cooked starches such as tubers provided the brains of our ancestors with higher amounts of blood glucose, which fueled the expansion of brain matter. To this point, researchers from the University of Florence in Italy recently discovered oat residue on a 32,000-year-old Paleolithic grinding tool, meaning our ancestors also thought oatmeal does a body good. Of course, you'd be wise to you stick mostly with less-processed forms of carbs in your diet such as sweet potatoes, whole grains, and whole fruit rather than more processed, less nutrient-dense options like loaves of doughy white bread.

You'll also want to shy away from an overabundance of protein and fat for the same digestive reasons. This makes a turkey drumstick or chili cheese fries not exactly optimal pre-workout fuel. However, a little bit of fat could provide a fuel source for your muscles, thereby helping reserve more carbohydrates for top-end efforts. A moderate amount of fat and protein can also serve to lower the glycemic load of your pre-workout eats and can stave off hunger. Some science also suggests that consuming protein before a workout can reduce the amount of muscular breakdown in response to training, which could serve to improve recovery and better maintain and build lean body mass.

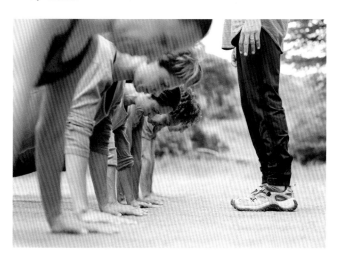

KNOW YOUR WORKOUT

What and how much you eat before exercise should depend on the type of workout you are planning. If a full day in the saddle or a 90-minute training session is on tap, you can gravitate toward more calories and higher intakes of carbohydrates since you'll be torching plenty of energy. For workouts that are focused on resistance training and strength-building exercises, it can be optimal to add more protein into your pre-workout fuel at the expense of some carbs to help limit muscle damage. For a typical lower-intensity gym workout that won't last much longer than an hour, a light snack of around 150 calories should be sufficient to keep you energized, as long as you consumed a well-balanced meal a couple of hours beforehand. This can also apply to athletes who are preparing for exercise that involves only a short bout of intense activity, such as sprint training.

SIP AND CHEW

It's never a good idea to start a workout with a water deficit, even if your workout is relegated to the weight room and not a steamy outdoor amphitheater. A *Journal of Applied Physiology* study found that dehydrated weight lifters produced higher levels of the stress hormone cortisol and lower levels of the muscle-building hormone testosterone in response to exercise, which can have a net effect of muscle breakdown.

So be sure to consume fluids such as water or tea on a regular basis through the day, and consider adding a cup or two of fluid to your pre-workout routine, especially if you are exercising first thing in the morning, as you'll likely awake dehydrated. Prehydration is also especially important if you are prone to sweating buckets or are about to tackle a workout in the heat. Fluid also serves the added function of helping with the digestion of the pre-workout food you eat.

Keep in mind that fruits also provide a source of hydration, and items such as the Watermelon Slushy (p. 67) and Maté Ginger Elixir (p. 68) serve an added purpose of flooding your body with hydrating fluid. However, you don't want to guzzle gallons of water before a workout in an attempt to hydrate, as you may end up with an uncomfortable water belly. So do your best to spread out your fluid intake.

SNACK ATTACK

Ready to sweat? Want to get the most out of your workout? Need a pre-workout snack, stat? This chapter delivers recipes that are designed to help the time-crunched, nutrition-conscious athlete prepare to outgun the competition by achieving the most effective training session or race possible.

That's because the pre-exercise food and drinks that follow are designed to deliver a steady release of energy or fluid needed for optimal performance to help you stay strong to the finish without bogging you down. And since many of the recipes such as the Beet Yogurt Bowl (p. 39) require little more than the assembly of some make-ahead items, they are also a perfect way to hack your pre-training routine by being ready when you are. This chapter is also your go-to source for some great options if you're traveling to an event and want to bring along some familiar items. Case in point: The Instant Porridge options (p. 36) can easily be prepared with nothing more than hot water in a hotel room. The Stuffed Dates (p. 44) can be nibbled as you drive to a race. Taking them along helps keep your pre-race fueling consistent with your training so you're not fretting about what to eat and instead are focusing more mental energy on the task ahead.

Perhaps most important, you'll be delighted to now have many more fuel options than the standard packaged energy bar, bowl of cereal, or peanut butter spread on toast. Just the thought of biting into the

Orange Crush Power Bites (p. 52) or spooning up some Java Chia Pudding (p. 41) makes me motivated to stop punching the keyboard and head out the door. The fact that they are healthy is a bonus and makes them perfect for everyday snacking. Simply mix them up at the drop of a hat to provide stamina on demand. Game on!

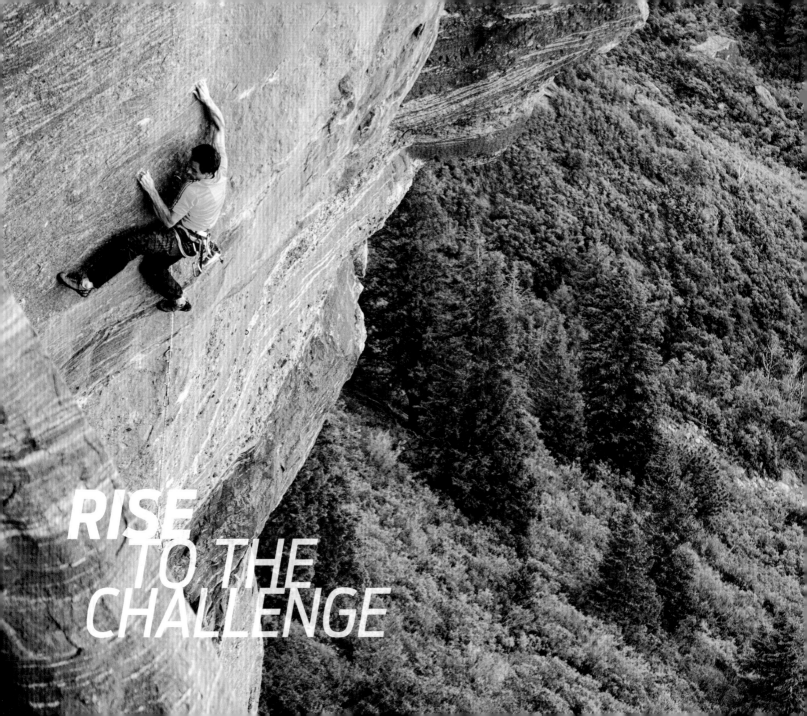

RISE
TO THE
CHALLENGE

RECIPES FOR **BEFORE**

D Dairy-free   **F** Freezer-friendly   **G** Gluten-free   **P** Paleo-friendly   **V** Vegetarian or vegan-friendly

Look to the Game Changers section to find simple substitutions that make nearly every recipe more friendly for specific diets.

APPLE SWEET POTATO MASH

High in complex carbohydrates, the sweet spud can provide some long-lasting energy for your impending exercise pursuit. But there's no need to put your workout on hold while you roast or boil one up when this nifty microwave mash gets the job done quickly. Some add-ins, such as maple syrup, applesauce, and crunchy pumpkin seeds, provide more motivation to work out.

D G P V

SERVINGS: 1
ACTIVE TIME: 10 min.

Although digestion rates vary, you'll likely perform better if you give yourself 30 minutes or more for digestion.

1 medium-sized sweet potato, peeled and cubed
⅓ cup plain applesauce
2 teaspoons pure maple syrup
¼ teaspoon ground allspice
¼ teaspoon ground ginger (optional)
1 tablespoon raisins
1 tablespoon raw shelled pumpkin seeds (pepitas)

Place sweet potato cubes and 1 tablespoon water in a microwave-safe bowl. Cover with plastic wrap and poke a few holes in plastic to allow for venting. Microwave on high for 6 minutes, or until potato is fork-tender. The bowl will be very hot, so use oven mitts or a dish towel to remove from microwave.

Add applesauce, maple syrup, allspice, and ground ginger (if using) to bowl and mash together. Top with raisins and pumpkin seeds.

GAME CHANGERS Replace applesauce with pear sauce + Mash in cinnamon instead of allspice + Use dried cranberries instead of raisins + Swap out pumpkin seeds for sunflower seeds

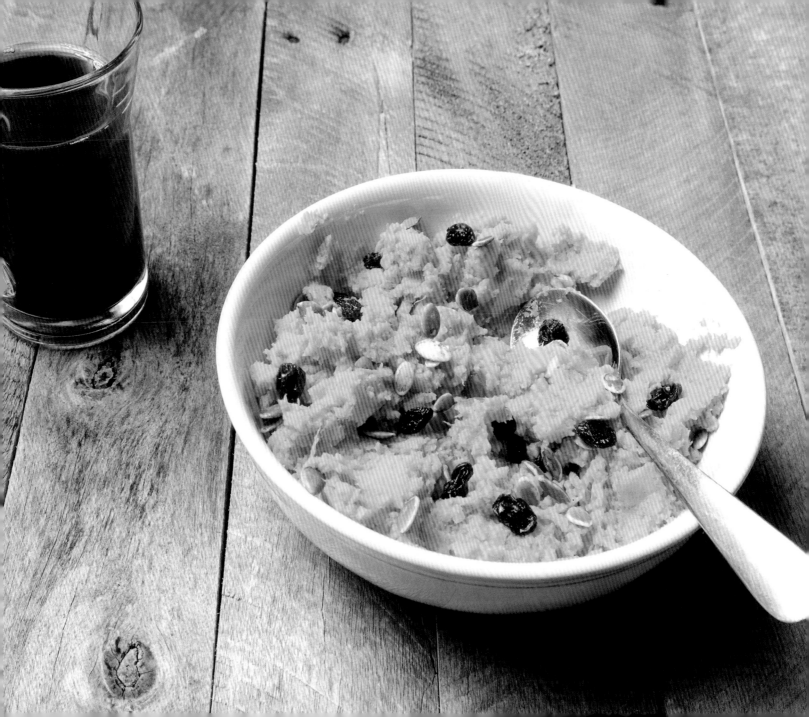

INSTANT PORRIDGE

A bowl of steamy porridge is pre-workout comfort food that provides some stick-to-your-ribs energy without feeling heavy. Don't settle for the lackluster instant porridge from a packet, because making your own couldn't be simpler. These pre-assembled instant oatmeals are great for camping and backpacking trips, as well as before clocking a long run or bike ride. Of course, you can also turn to them when in need of a lightning-fast breakfast to kick-start an active day.

D G V

SERVINGS: 4
ACTIVE TIME: 15 min.

Additive-free freeze-dried fruit is made by simply sucking out the water in the fruit to leave behind a shelf-stable, crunchy, sweet snack. It's perfect in DIY instant porridge because it rehydrates quickly and tastes as good as fresh fruit. If you can't find packages in stores, try online sources like www.nuts.com.

For a creamier porridge, mix in 1 tablespoon dry milk powder before adding the hot water.

1⅓ cups quick-cook oats
(not larger-flake rolled oats)

PB&J

⅓ cup powdered peanut butter, such as PB2
½ ounce freeze-dried strawberries (about ⅓ cup)
2–3 tablespoons coconut sugar or brown sugar
⅛ teaspoon salt

APPLE CINNAMON

1 ounce apple chips, roughly chopped (about ⅔ cup)
⅓ cup thinly sliced pecans
2–3 tablespoons coconut sugar, brown sugar, or maple sugar
¾ teaspoon cinnamon
⅛ teaspoon salt

CURRY CASHEW

⅓ cup roughly chopped unsalted roasted cashews
¼ cup golden raisins
3 tablespoons unsweetened shredded coconut
2–3 tablespoons coconut sugar or brown sugar
2 teaspoons yellow curry powder
⅛ teaspoon salt

MOCHA

⅓ cup roughly chopped hazelnuts
1 ounce freeze-dried banana (not banana chips), roughly chopped (about ½ cup)
2–3 tablespoons coconut sugar or brown sugar
1 tablespoon unsweetened cocoa powder
2 teaspoons instant espresso powder
½ teaspoon cinnamon
⅛ teaspoon salt

APRICOT GINGER

⅓ cup chopped dried apricots
⅓ cup chopped or unsalted dry-roasted almonds
1 teaspoon ground ginger
½ teaspoon ground allspice
2–3 tablespoons coconut sugar or brown sugar
⅛ teaspoon salt

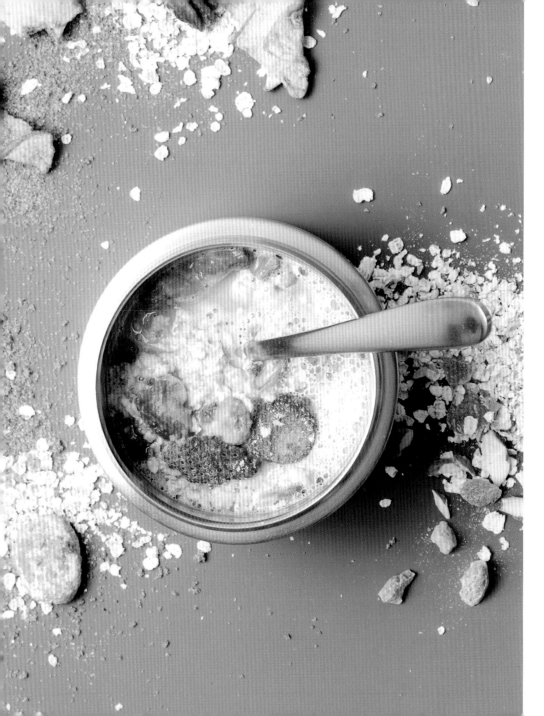

Preheat oven to 350ºF. Spread oats on a rimmed baking sheet and bake until they turn golden and smell toasted, about 12 minutes, stirring once halfway through cooking time. The oats can go from toasted to burnt quickly, so mind the oven. Let cool and then combine with one of the flavor mixes and store in a glass jar or divide among four sandwich-sized zip-top bags until ready to use.

To make a bowl of porridge, place about ½ cup of an oat mixture in a bowl and top with ½ to ¾ cup boiling water, depending on desired consistency. Stir, cover, and let soak for 2 to 3 minutes. To prepare in microwave, top ½ cup oat mixture with ½ to ¾ cup water and microwave on high for about 1 minute. For transport, transfer the oat mixture and boiled water to a food-grade thermos.

GAME CHANGERS Use oats labeled "gluten-free" or replace the oats with quinoa, spelt, or Kamut flakes

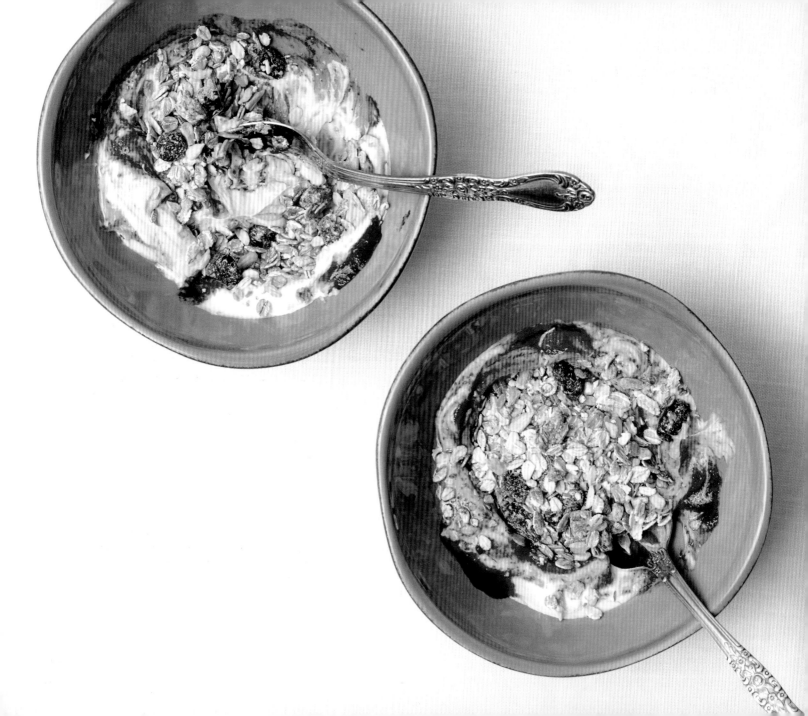

BEET YOGURT BOWL

Beets have been linked to performance-related benefits courtesy of their blood vessel–widening nitrates. But this recipe shows that you can do more than just drink them in juice form as part of your pre-workout dietary routine. This beet puree takes on a rich and sweet personality that, when paired with easy-to-digest yogurt, makes for a bowlful of nutritional greatness. In fact, a recent study out of the Australian Institute of Sport found that dairy consumption among cyclists before a 90-minute ride had no negative impact on gut comfort or performance. But you can use a dairy-free yogurt such as coconut if needed. The muesli from the Muesli Salad (p. 193) works wonderfully as a topping, and so do blackberries, pomegranate seeds, or chopped mango.

D G P V

SERVINGS: 6
ACTIVE TIME: 15 min.

Roasting beets brings out their natural sweetness, but you can also steam or boil them. Some grocers even now carry precooked beets.

1 pound beets, ends trimmed and chopped into chunks
2 teaspoons canola, grapeseed, or light olive oil
1¼ cups coconut milk beverage
   Juice of ½ lime
2 tablespoons honey
1 tablespoon coconut oil (optional)
2 teaspoons chopped fresh ginger
½ teaspoon cinnamon
⅛ teaspoon salt
3 cups plain low-fat yogurt
1½ cups granola or muesli of choice

Preheat oven to 400°F. Place beets on a baking sheet and toss with oil. Roast until tender, stirring once, about 35 minutes. Let beets cool.

Place beets in a blender along with coconut milk, lime juice, honey, coconut oil (if using), ginger, cinnamon, and salt; blend until smooth. The mixture should be fairly thick, but add a touch more coconut milk if needed to help with blending. Chill mixture until needed, for up to 10 days.

When ready to serve, place ½ cup yogurt in a bowl and swirl in about ⅓ cup beet puree. Top with ¼ cup granola or muesli and a drizzle of additional honey, if desired.

GAME CHANGERS Swap out lime juice for lemon juice + Blend in maple syrup or agave syrup instead of honey + For grain-free, top with chopped nuts or seeds instead of granola

RASPBERRY CHIA PUDDING

Aztec and Incan warriors of days gone by reportedly ate chia for strength and stamina during battle. The tiny seed is also a go-to fuel source for the Tarahumara, a tribe of super-runners in Mexico. Why? The soluble fiber in chia is thought to form a gel in your gut, as it does when mixed with liquids such as almond milk, ensuring a more steady release of energy during a workout. Chia's renaissance as a superfood also stems from its range of important nutrients, including heart-healthy omega-3 fats. And unlike flax, which contains a harder outer shell, chia does not need to be ground for the body to access its nutritional payload. For that reason, this pudding is also a stellar option for an ultra-healthy dessert.

D G P V

SERVINGS: 2
ACTIVE TIME: 10 min.

If you're sensitive to fiber before a workout, be sure to give yourself some extra time between eating this pudding and lacing up your shoes.

1½ cups plain almond milk
1 cup fresh or frozen, thawed raspberries
1 tablespoon fresh lemon juice
1 tablespoon honey
1 teaspoon vanilla extract
¼ cup chia seeds
2 tablespoons cacao nibs (optional)

Place almond milk, raspberries, lemon juice, honey, and vanilla in a blender and blend until smooth. Divide mixture between two jars. Add 2 tablespoons chia seeds to each jar, seal shut, and give the jars a good shake. Chill for at least 3 hours and up to 3 days. Serve topped with cacao nibs, if desired.

GAME CHANGERS Replace almond milk with other milks such as hemp, cashew, or even cow + Use strawberries instead of raspberries + Add ½ teaspoon almond extract instead of vanilla extract

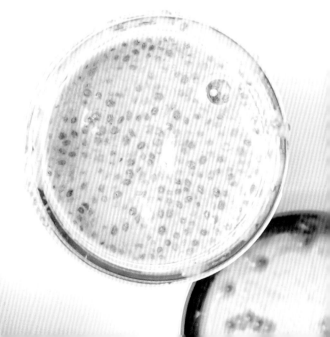

JAVA CHIA PUDDING

This pudding's dynamic duo of chia and coffee is sure to lift your workout to new heights. A 2011 study published in the *Journal of Strength and Conditioning Research* found that athletes who included nutrient-dense chia in their pre-workout fueling experienced a boost in running performance. On top of that, the caffeine from coffee will deliver a little extra lift. You can also blend in some protein powder and make this pudding post-training worthy.

SERVINGS: 2
ACTIVE TIME: 10 min.

Stirring in the chia seeds after blending keeps them whole and more absorbent so that you end up with a thicker texture.

¾ cup cooled brewed coffee
¾ cup plain almond milk
2 tablespoons pure maple syrup
1 tablespoon unsweetened cocoa powder
1 tablespoon nut butter
1 teaspoon vanilla extract
½ teaspoon ground cardamom
⅔ cup chopped fresh or frozen cherries
¼ cup chia seeds

Place all of the ingredients except for the chia seeds and cherries in a blender and blend until smooth.

Divide mixture between two jars. Add half of the cherries and chia seeds to each jar, seal shut, and give the jars a good shake. Chill for at least 3 hours or up to 3 days.

GAME CHANGERS Blend in coconut milk beverage or cow milk instead of almond milk + Swap out nut butter for a seed butter such as sunflower + Season with cinnamon instead of cardamom + Stir in dried tart cherries instead of using fresh or frozen

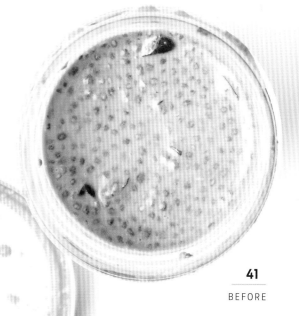

MAPLE MILLET PUDDING

Before lacing up for some serious calorie-burning, spoon up a bowl of this whole-grain pudding. Similar to more traditional rice pudding, this one, made with gluten-free millet, is full of slow-burning carbohydrate energy. Serve it straight from the fridge or enjoy it warm with a splash of additional milk. You can add a sprinkling of nuts, seeds, fresh berries, or dried fruit such as tart cherries. I also often add a small drizzle of additional maple syrup.

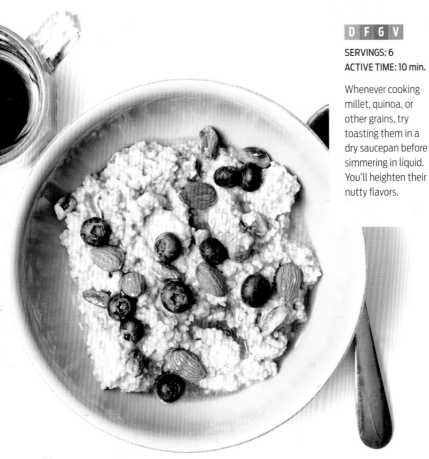

D F G V

SERVINGS: 6
ACTIVE TIME: 10 min.

Whenever cooking millet, quinoa, or other grains, try toasting them in a dry saucepan before simmering in liquid. You'll heighten their nutty flavors.

¾ cup millet
3½ cups unsweetened almond milk
¼ cup pure maple syrup
1 teaspoon vanilla extract
1 teaspoon cinnamon
¼ teaspoon nutmeg

Place millet in a medium-sized dry saucepan and heat over medium until it begins to pop and smell fragrant, about 3 minutes, stirring often. Stir in milk, maple syrup, vanilla, cinnamon, nutmeg, and a pinch of salt.

Bring mixture to a light boil, reduce heat to low, and simmer, covered, stirring occasionally, until millet is cooked through and mixture has thickened, about 25 minutes. Remove from heat and let cool in pan to room temperature. The pudding will thicken further as it cools. Keep chilled for up to 5 days.

GAME CHANGERS Use low-fat cow milk, rice milk, or coconut milk beverage instead of almond milk **+** Swap out cinnamon for ¾ teaspoon ground cardamom

RICE CON LECHE

Got a long way to ride or run? Fuel up on this slow-burning tropical riff on rice pudding. Slightly sweet with a great chew, Chinese black rice (also sold under the name Forbidden Rice) could very well be my favorite grain. Studies show that it also harbors high levels of the same potent anthocyanin antioxidants found in dark berries such as blueberries. So I often cook up a batch big enough to make this dish and have leftover rice for salads and stir-fries. You can also add a dusting of cinnamon before serving.

D G V

SERVINGS: 1
ACTIVE TIME: 10 min.

Not to be confused with canned coconut milk, coconut milk beverage in a carton is designed to have a mouthfeel that is more similar to regular milk. It's also not nearly as high in fat as full-fat coconut milk, making it a better choice shortly before a workout. It's great in smoothies, too.

½ cup coconut milk beverage
1 teaspoon honey
½ cup cooked black rice
½ cup cubed mango
1 tablespoon chopped cashews

Heat coconut milk and honey in a small saucepan to just under a boil, or microwave in a microwave-safe bowl for about 40 seconds, until warmed through.

Place cooked rice in a serving bowl and pour coconut milk on top. Scatter on mango and cashews.

GAME CHANGERS Try cashew milk in lieu of coconut milk + Replace mango with pineapple + Use pumpkin seeds instead of cashews

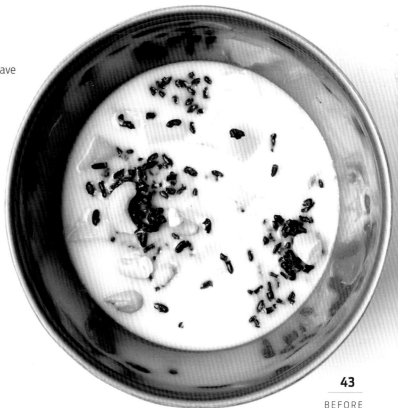

STUFFED DATES

The natural sugars in soft and succulent Medjool dates offer a concentrated shot of carbohydrate energy before a workout so you're ready to shine straight from the starting blocks. Dates also provide potassium, which aids in muscle functioning. Stuff them with these fillings and it's guaranteed that you'll have this pre-exercise nibble in heavy rotation after the first bite.

D G P V

SERVINGS: 8
ACTIVE TIME: 15 min.

Coconut butter is made by pureeing coconut flesh into a buttery spread consistency (as opposed to squeezing out the fat from the coconut flesh, which produces coconut oil). Coconut butter is great for stuffing into dates or slathering on morning toast for a taste of the tropics.

16 Medjool dates (about ¾ pound)

CITRUS RICOTTA

½ cup part-skim ricotta cheese
2 teaspoons orange zest
1 teaspoon vanilla extract

OPEN SESAME

½ cup tahini (sesame paste)
Zest of 1 lemon

COCONUT ZING

⅓ cup coconut butter (not coconut oil)
1 teaspoon ground ginger

Stir together one of the ingredient combinations. Using a knife, slice an opening in the dates (without cutting them in half) and remove the pit. Gently pry open dates with fingers, and spoon in the filling. Keep chilled in an airtight container for up to 5 days.

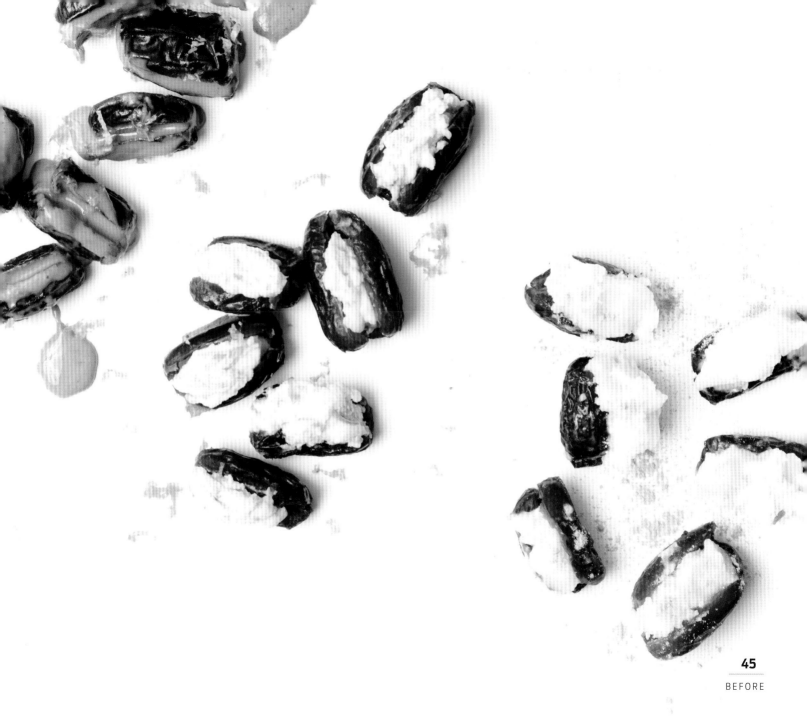

CHOCOLATE BANANA LETTUCE WRAPS

If starch before a workout leaves you feeling sluggish, try this fresh approach to a wrap. It's ideal for when you're in a pre-exercise rush. For some crunch, add a sprinkle of granola.

D G P V SERVINGS: 1 | ACTIVE TIME: 5 min.

1 large Boston or butter lettuce leaf*
1 tablespoon chocolate hazelnut butter
1 small banana
1 teaspoon honey

* *Use a mild-tasting lettuce*

Spread chocolate hazelnut butter on one side of the lettuce leaf. Top with banana, drizzle on honey, and fold over the leaf.

GAME CHANGERS Spread on almond, peanut, or cashew butter instead of chocolate hazelnut ✦ Try apple slices instead of banana ✦ Use maple syrup or agave instead of honey

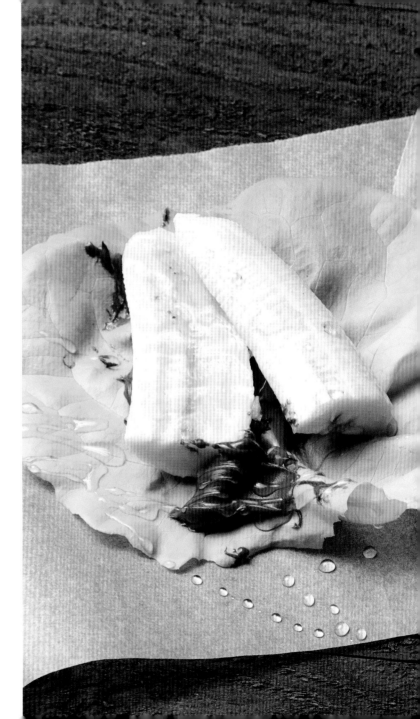

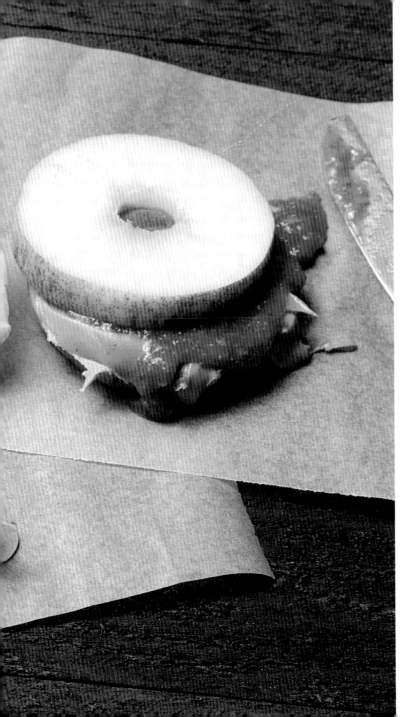

APPLE SANDWICHES

This riff on iconic PB&J is great for both gym bags and lunch boxes. The dynamic duo of apple and figs provides carbs to give you the little rev your body needs. You can add extra crunch by sprinkling on some granola.

D G P V   SERVINGS: 6 | ACTIVE TIME: 15 min.

½ cup dried figs, stems removed

¼ teaspoon cinnamon

1 teaspoon grated fresh ginger

1 teaspoon lemon zest

3 tablespoons peanut butter or other nut butter

2 large apples, cored and sliced into six ¼-inch-thick rounds*

* If not eating right away, you can brush the apple slices with a solution of 3 tablespoons water and 1 tablespoon lemon juice to slow browning.

Place figs in a bowl, cover with 1 cup boiling water, and let soak 30 minutes. Place figs, the soaking liquid, cinnamon, ginger, lemon zest, and a pinch of salt in a blender and blend until slightly chunky. Let cool. Jam can be chilled for up to 10 days.

Spread about 1½ teaspoons nut butter and 1 tablespoon fig jam on one apple slice and top with another apple slice. Repeat with remaining apple slices and filling as needed.

GAME CHANGERS   Use store-bought berry jam or cherry preserves instead of the fig mixture + Replace nut butter with coconut butter or seed butter

GRAHAM CRACKER
PUMPKIN BUTTER SMASH

Good for more than s'mores, graham crackers are a great vehicle for transporting this velvety pumpkin butter into your body for a shot of pre-workout carbs. You can now even find gluten-free graham crackers. These can also work for fueling as you push the pace during a workout, but keep in mind that the crackers won't stay crispy for very long once the pumpkin butter is applied.

D F G V

SERVINGS: 8
ACTIVE TIME: 15 min.

Extra pumpkin butter can be frozen in an airtight container for up to 1 month. It's also great smeared on toast and apple slices or even mixed into warm oatmeal.

1 (14-ounce) can pure pumpkin puree
⅓ cup brown sugar
⅓ cup apple cider
½ teaspoon ground ginger
½ teaspoon cinnamon
¼ teaspoon ground cloves
¼ teaspoon nutmeg
1 teaspoon vanilla extract
1 tablespoon fresh lemon juice
32 graham crackers

Place pumpkin, sugar, cider, ginger, cinnamon, cloves, and nutmeg in a medium-sized saucepan. Bring to a boil over medium-high heat, reduce heat to medium-low, and simmer until the mixture is thickened, about 30 minutes. Stir the pumpkin butter frequently during cooking and keep the lid slightly ajar to help steam escape yet still avoid splatter—a wooden spoon handle can help with this. Stir in vanilla, lemon juice, and a pinch of salt. Let pumpkin butter cool to room temperature. Transfer to a container and keep chilled for up to 2 weeks.

To serve, spread some pumpkin butter on a graham cracker and top with another cracker.

GAME CHANGERS Try pureed butternut squash instead of pumpkin ✦ Stir in apple juice in place of apple cider ✦ Use store-bought pumpkin pie spice instead of the spices ✦ Use gluten-free graham crackers

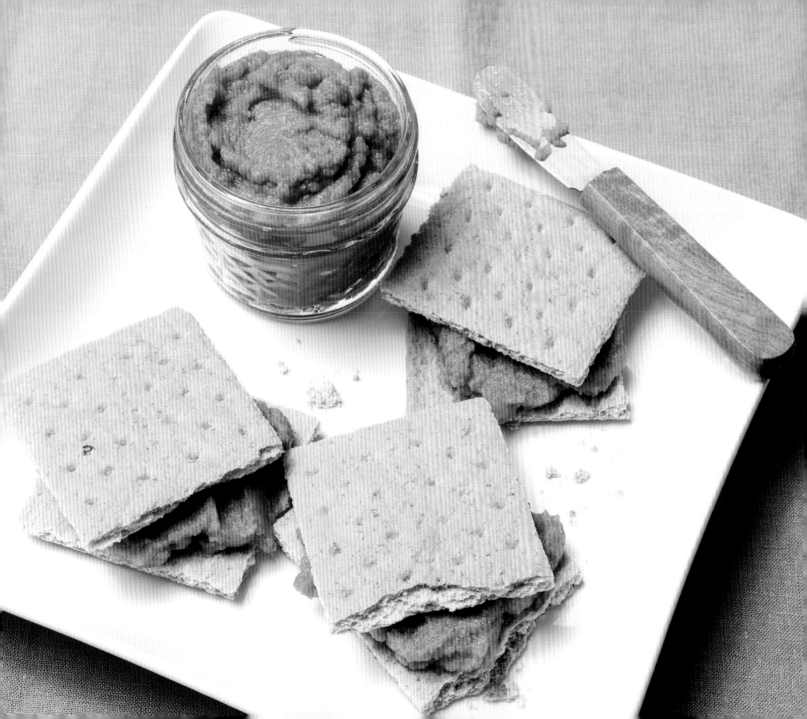

OPEN-FACED RICE CAKE SANDWICHES

On their own, rice cakes are about as exciting as C-SPAN. But the crunchy, easy-to-digest rounds are just as versatile as toast for piling on all sorts of great flavors to help you rise to the occasion. And this pre-workout nosh is ready in about the same amount of time it takes to lace up your sneakers.

SERVINGS: 4
ACTIVE TIME: 5 min.

I suggest sticking with plain varieties of rice cakes since flavored ones often include ingredients that sound like they belong more in a laboratory than in your stomach.

4 plain rice cakes

BACK IN BLACK
SPREAD*
1 cup plain Greek yogurt
1 teaspoon vanilla extract
1 teaspoon orange zest or lemon zest

TOPPING
1 cup blackberries
4 teaspoons honey or pure maple syrup

* *Stir ingredients together in a small bowl before applying.*

BLUEBERRY CHEESECAKE
SPREAD
¼ cup peanut butter

TOPPING
⅔ cup plain whipped cream cheese
½ cup fresh blueberries
2 teaspoons honey

BERRY HUMMUS
SPREAD
½ cup prepared hummus

TOPPING
¼ cup dried cranberries

NUTTY PEAR
SPREAD
¼ cup almond butter

TOPPING
2 small pears, thinly sliced
2 ounces soft goat cheese, crumbled (about ½ cup)

Apply an equal amount of the spread and topping to each cake.

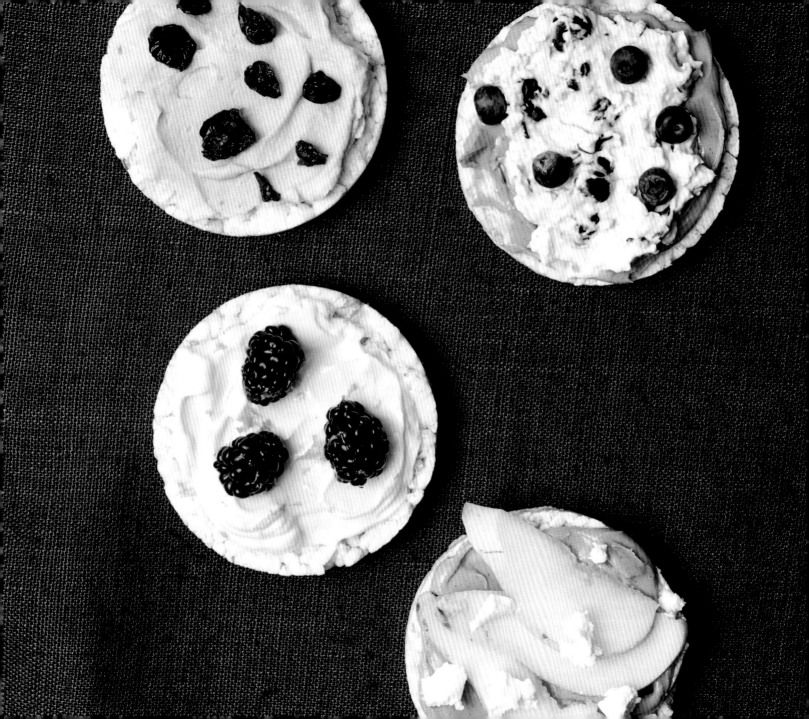

ORANGE CRUSH POWER BITES

These great balls of nutrition are ridiculously easy to make, and you'll have plenty on hand when a hard workout is fast approaching or you're in need of a less hazardous late-night nibble than a bag of chips. The bit of fat in these will help slow the release of sugar into your bloodstream, a benefit that can help prevent the spike-and-crash in blood sugar that can occur in some people during the initial stages of exercise when they eat high-glycemic carbs such as gels close to game time.

D F G P V

SERVINGS: 8
ACTIVE TIME: 20 min.

Although it may sound counterintuitive, studies suggest that people who regularly crunch on high-calorie nuts are more likely to maintain healthier body weights. It's thought that the synergy of protein, fiber, healthy fats, antioxidants, and minerals in nuts such as pecans and walnuts can help keep you svelte.

1 large carrot, peeled and roughly chopped
½ cup pecans
½ cup walnuts
1 cup dried apricots
  Zest of 1 medium orange
2 teaspoons minced fresh ginger
½ teaspoon cinnamon
¼ teaspoon nutmeg
¼ teaspoon ground cloves
⅛ teaspoon salt
⅓ cup unsweetened shredded coconut

Place carrot, pecans, and walnuts in a food processor and pulse until pulverized. Add apricots, orange zest, ginger, cinnamon, nutmeg, cloves, and salt and blend until mixture sticks together when pressed between your fingers.

Roll mixture between your hands into 1-inch balls. You should have about 16 balls. Place coconut on a plate and roll balls in the coconut, pressing down gently to adhere. Chill in an airtight container for up to 1 week.

GAME CHANGERS Use almonds instead of pecans + Swap out orange zest for lemon zest + Replace coconut with hemp seeds or sesame seeds

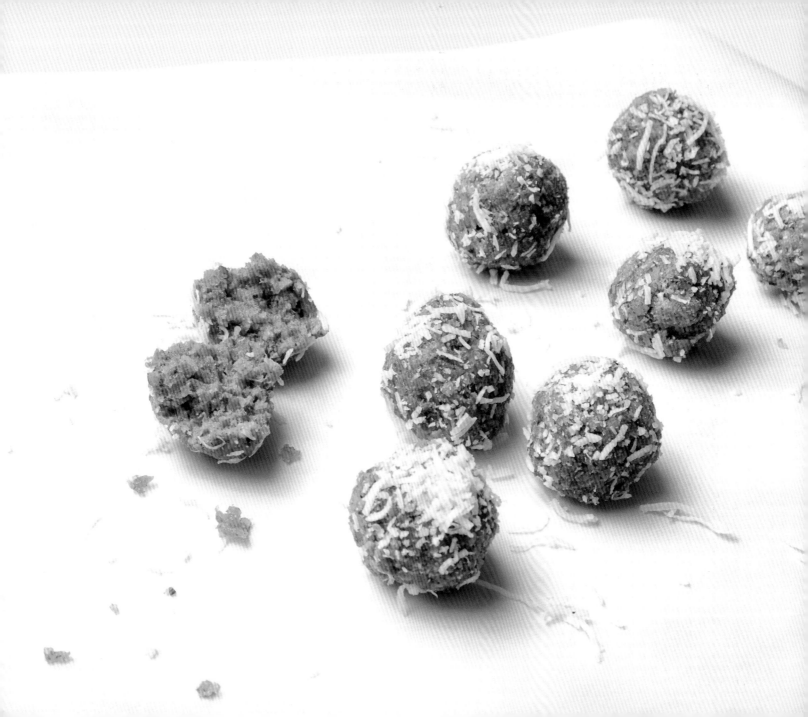

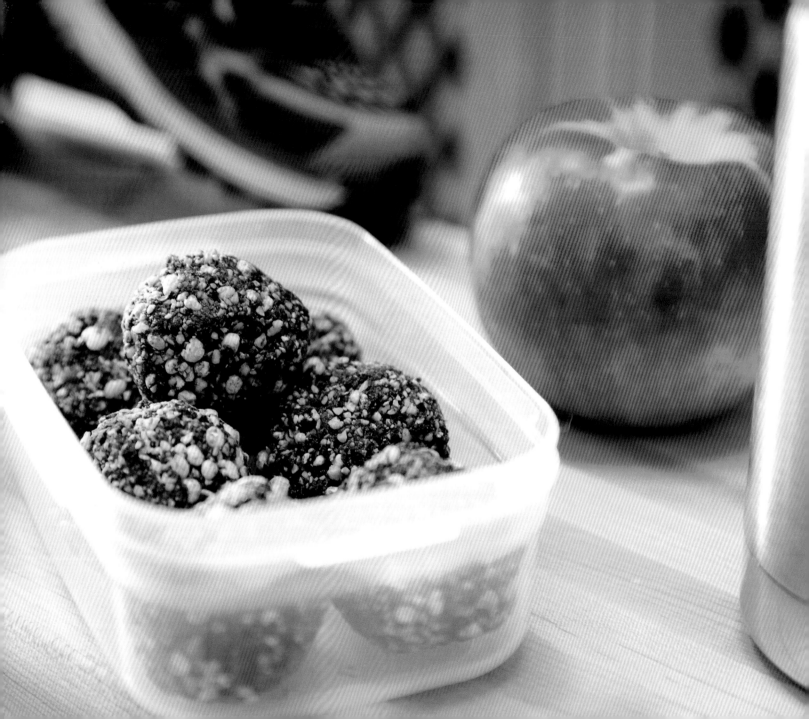

CHOCOLATE QUINOA ENERGY BALLS

There is a good reason why energy balls like this chocolaty incarnation remain one of the most popular DIY fuel options for athletes. They can provide a tasty instant hit of energy when you need it most—whether it's before breaking a sweat or during exercise. They're also great as a snack at the office to dampen vending machine temptation. You can take these balls into different flavor directions: Add some zing with orange zest or blend in a touch of chili powder for a Mayan taste. And of course, cinnamon can only make anything with chocolate better. Or go even more decadent and pulse in ½ cup of dark chocolate chips along with the quinoa.

D F G V

SERVINGS: 8
ACTIVE TIME: 20 min.

Puffed quinoa is simply quinoa that has been puffed (popped) using heat to give it a crisp texture. Look for it at natural food stores or in the health food section of larger grocers among other boxed cereal and also in bulk-food bins.

1 cup raw almonds
1 cup pitted dried plums (aka prunes)
¼ cup unsweetened cocoa powder
2 tablespoons almond butter
2 tablespoons honey
1 cup puffed quinoa

Place almonds in a food processor and blend until almonds resemble coarse sand. Add plums, cocoa powder, almond butter, honey, and a couple pinches of salt. Blend until the mixture sticks together when pressed between your fingers. Pulse in puffed quinoa.

Form mixture into 1-inch balls. You should have about 16 balls. Keep chilled in an airtight container for up to 1 week.

GAME CHANGERS Use pecans or walnuts instead of almonds ✦ Swap out dried plums for pitted Medjool dates ✦ Replace honey with agave syrup or brown rice syrup ✦ Pulse in puffed millet instead of puffed quinoa

MUESLI SQUARES

Easier and quicker than most bar recipes, these squares can help crush any pre-workout hunger pangs. I find that they're easy to digest and don't give me any GI problems, making them safe to eat just before your workout. Gluten-free versions of muesli such as Bob's Red Mill are now available. You can also make up a bigger batch of the muesli recipe from the Muesli Salad (p. 193) and use that here.

D F G V

SERVINGS: 12
ACTIVE TIME: 20 min.

To make it easier to mold parchment paper to your pan, simply scrunch up a piece of parchment and run water over it. Squeeze out the excess water and press the paper into the pan.

1 (13.5-ounce) can light coconut milk
1 large egg
2 tablespoons melted and cooled coconut oil
2 teaspoons vanilla extract
1 teaspoon ground allspice
¼ teaspoon salt
2½ cups muesli of choice
1 large banana, finely chopped

Preheat oven to 350°F. Line an 8 × 8–inch square baking pan with a piece of parchment paper large enough so that about 1 inch overhangs the edges.

In a large bowl, whisk together coconut milk, egg, coconut oil, vanilla, allspice, and salt. Stir in muesli and banana.

Pour mixture into pan and bake for 40 minutes, or until set and edges begin to darken. Let cool completely in pan and then carefully lift out the muesli mixture using the parchment overhang. Slice into 12 squares. Store for up to 5 days in an airtight container with a piece of parchment paper separating the layers of bars.

GAME CHANGERS Season with cinnamon in lieu of allspice ✚ Use store-bought granola instead of muesli ✚ Replace the banana with a plantain

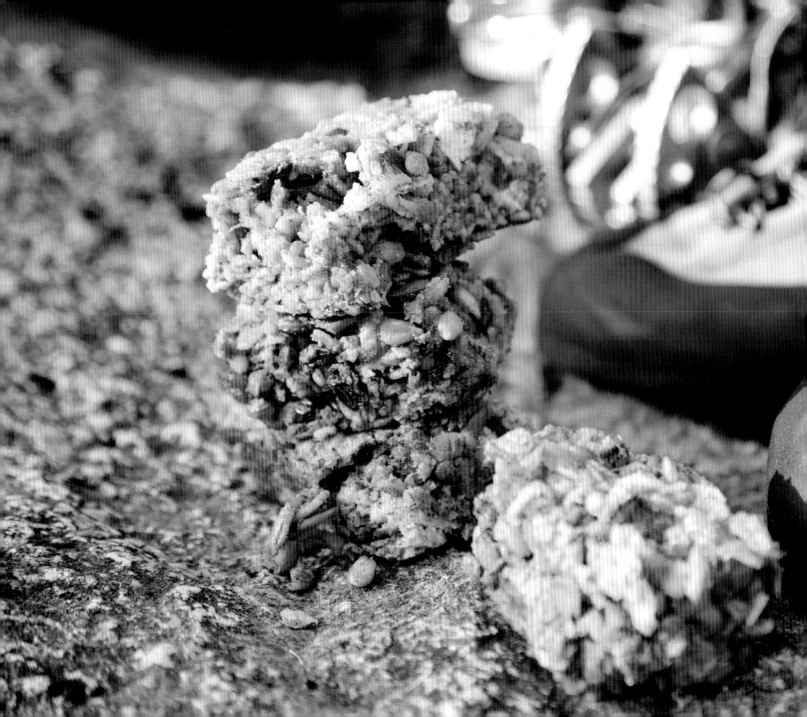

PUMPKIN DATE MUFFINS

The one-two punch of pumpkin and dates means these rustic muffins don't require any sugar to sweeten your pre-workout fueling. They're a great option when you need a snack that you can take with you to the office for when you're planning to bolt straight from work to the gym or a group ride. These will be moister, and unapologetically more rustic, than your typical muffin, so it's best to store them in the refrigerator once they've cooled.

D F G V

SERVINGS: 12
ACTIVE TIME: 20 min.

Milled from lower-gluten soft wheat, whole wheat pastry flour produces less-heavy baked goods than does regular whole wheat flour, which is ground from hard wheat. Look for it at stores with well-stocked baking sections or order online at places such as www.bobsredmill.com.

1 cup roughly pitted dried dates
1 cup canned pure pumpkin puree
⅓ cup melted coconut oil
2 teaspoons vanilla extract
1 large egg
1¾ cups whole wheat pastry flour
⅓ cup ground flaxseed
1 teaspoon baking powder
¼ teaspoon baking soda
1 teaspoon cinnamon
½ teaspoon nutmeg
¼ teaspoon salt
½ cup chopped walnuts

Place dates in a bowl and cover with 1 cup boiling water and let soak about 20 minutes.

Preheat oven to 350°F. Combine dates, soaking liquid, pumpkin, oil, and vanilla in a blender or food processor and blend until smooth. Stir in egg.

In a large bowl, stir together flour, flaxseed, baking powder, baking soda, cinnamon, nutmeg, and salt. Add wet ingredients to dry ingredients and mix gently until everything is moist. Fold in walnuts.

Divide mixture among 12 standard-sized silicone muffin cups, or greased or paper-lined metal muffin cups. Bake for 22 minutes, or until a toothpick inserted in the center of a muffin comes out mostly clean. Let cool for a few minutes before unmolding and cooling completely, preferably on metal cooling racks. Muffins can be kept chilled for up to 5 days or frozen for up to 2 months.

GAME CHANGERS Use cooked and pureed butternut squash or sweet potato instead of pumpkin ✦ Swap out coconut oil for melted butter or a neutral-tasting oil such as grapeseed or canola ✦ Use all-purpose flour, spelt flour, or 1-to-1 gluten-free flour blend instead of whole wheat pastry flour

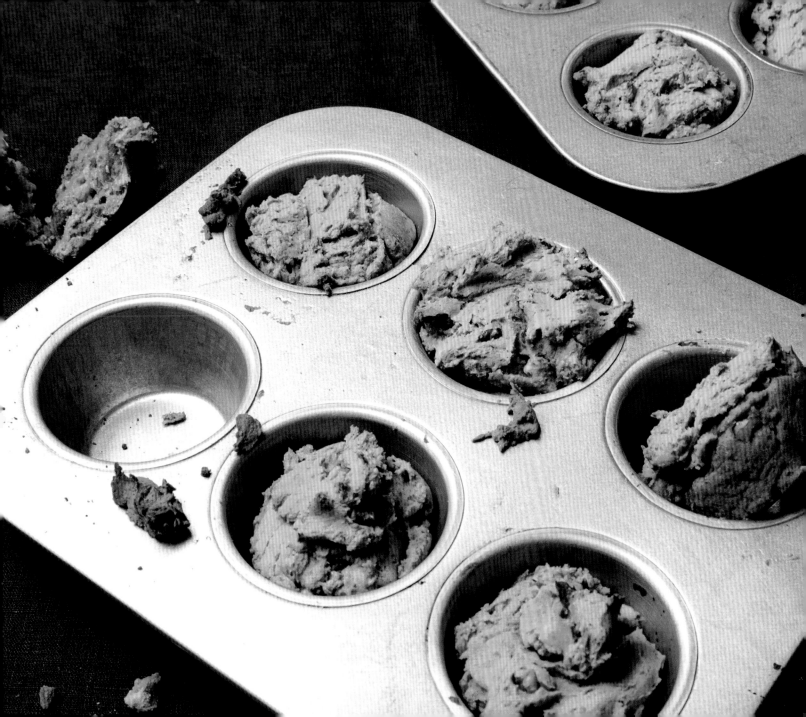

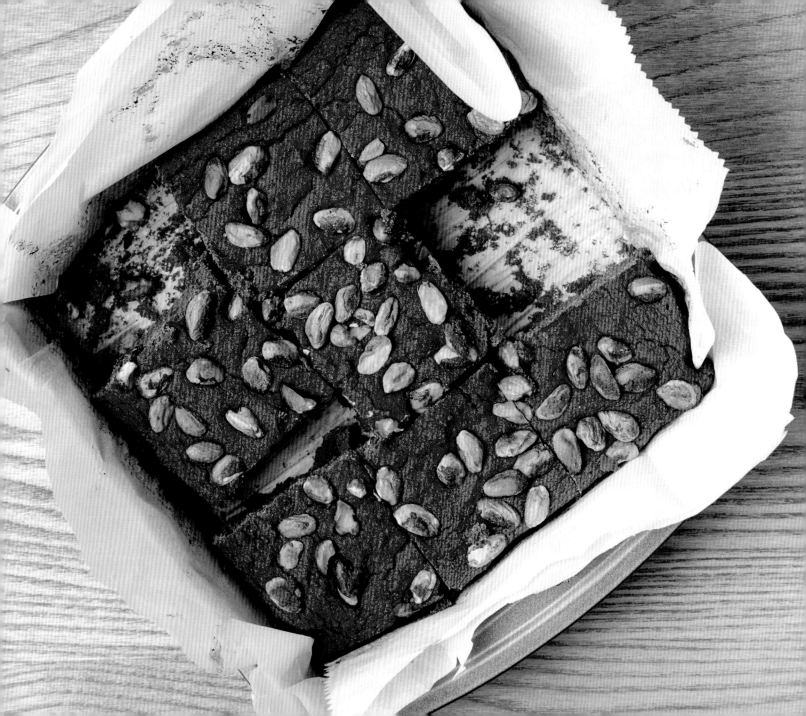

BEET PISTACHIO BARS

Juice isn't the only way to get your pre-workout beet power. Thanks to a carefully planned combination of ingredients, these tender bars aren't overly beety, making them a bright addition to your sports-nutrition plan. Taking the time to roast the beets helps coax out their natural sweetness. I've listed the chocolate chips as optional, but they always find a way to sneak into my bar batter. The scattering of pistachios on top offers up great crunch and added nutrition.

`D F G V`

SERVINGS: 9
ACTIVE TIME: 25 min.

Coconut oil is solid at room temperature. To melt for recipes, measure out the specified amount in a small bowl and microwave for 30 seconds or until liquefied. Or place in the oven as it preheats and allow the oven heat to melt the oil.

- 1 pound beets (about 4 medium-sized), peeled and chopped
- 2 teaspoons canola, grapeseed, or light olive oil
- ½ cup low-fat milk
- ½ cup brown sugar
- ⅓ cup melted coconut oil
- Zest of 1 lemon
- 2 large eggs
- 1 cup brown rice flour
- ¼ cup coconut flour
- 2 teaspoons baking powder
- 1 teaspoon cinnamon
- ½ teaspoon salt
- ½ cup dark chocolate chips (optional)
- ½ cup unsalted shelled pistachios

Preheat oven to 400°F. Place beets in an 8 × 8–inch square baking pan and toss with oil. Roast until tender, about 35 minutes.

Place roasted beets, milk, sugar, coconut oil, and lemon zest in a blender or food processor and blend until smooth. Blend in eggs.

In a large bowl, stir together rice flour, coconut flour, baking powder, cinnamon, and salt. Add wet ingredients to dry ingredients and mix gently until everything is moist. Fold in chocolate chips, if using.

Line the square baking pan used to roast the beets with parchment paper so there is at least a 1-inch overhang. Place beet mixture in pan in an even layer. Sprinkle pistachios on top and press down gently to help them adhere. Bake for 30 minutes, or until batter is set in the middle. Let cool completely in pan, then lift out using parchment overhang and slice into 9 squares. Keep chilled for up to 7 days.

GAME CHANGERS Replace milk with a plain nondairy milk such as almond + Swap out brown sugar for coconut or turbinado sugar + Use orange zest instead of lemon

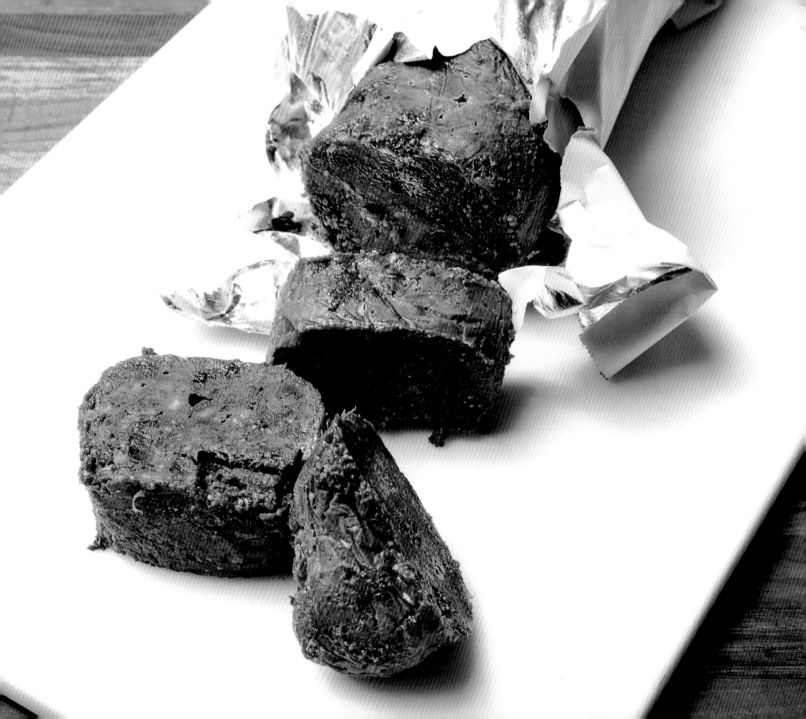

ESPRESSO FRUIT LOG

This bundle of fruity goodness won't freeze solid, so you can just slice and eat it straight from the freezer when you need a quick energy fix before feeling the burn. And here's more reason to embrace your inner Willy Wonka: British researchers found that eating dark chocolate products such as unsweetened cocoa powder and the antioxidant payload they contain before working out can lessen muscle oxidative stress in response to exercise—an indication of less muscular damage that can translate into better recovery. The addition of walnuts and protein powder serves to slow the release of the carbohydrates from the dried fruit for more sustained energy instead of a short burst and subsequent crash. You can also scatter some unsweetened shredded coconut on the plastic wrap and roll the fruit mixture in it.

D F G P V

SERVINGS: 8
ACTIVE TIME: 20 min.

If using the more expensive soft Medjool dates, they generally don't need to be soaked prior to blending.

My preference for the biggest antioxidant heft is to use raw cocoa powder, which is often spelled *cacao*.

2 tablespoons instant espresso powder

3 tablespoons unsweetened cocoa powder

1 cup pitted dates

1 cup dried figs, stems trimmed

½ cup walnut halves

½ cup raisins

⅓ cup protein powder

1 teaspoon cinnamon

1 teaspoon vanilla extract

Zest of 1 lemon (optional)

In a bowl, dissolve espresso powder and cocoa powder in ¼ cup boiling water. Let cool to room temperature. In a separate bowl, soak dates and figs in warm water for about 30 minutes. Drain and pat away excess moisture with a paper towel.

Place walnuts in a food processor and blend into small pieces. Add cocoa mixture, dates, figs, raisins, protein powder, cinnamon, vanilla, and lemon zest, if using. Blend until the mixture clumps together.

Place a large piece of plastic cling wrap on a cutting board and spoon the dried fruit mixture onto the bottom third of the plastic. Tightly roll the fruit mixture away from you sushi-style until it is wrapped in a couple layers of plastic. Place fruit roll in the freezer.

When ready for a pre-workout boost, simply peel back the plastic and slice away the desired amount of the log. Reroll and return to freezer for up to 1 month.

GAME CHANGERS Use hazelnuts or pecans instead of walnuts + Replace raisins with dried currants + Use orange zest in place of lemon zest

BLENDER BEET JUICE

Who would have thought that a root vegetable synonymous with borscht would turn out to be an effective performance-boosting aid? In research, naturally occurring nitrates in beets (also found in spinach!) help working muscles use oxygen more efficiently, resulting in improved performance. Beet juice is a great way to flood your body with nitrates quickly. But if you don't have a juicer or it's collecting dust behind the panini press because you hate the cleanup, this blender version means you're not out of luck.

D F G P V

SERVINGS: 2
ACTIVE TIME: 15 min.

I usually don't bother peeling my veggies—just give them a good scrubbing.

If you have a blender with a weak motor, you may want to use cooked beets. If using a juicer, simply omit the water.

If you like your juice thick, skip the straining step.

1 cup water
½ pound raw beets (about 2 medium-sized), trimmed and chopped
1 medium-sized apple, chopped
1 medium-sized carrot, chopped
1 cup spinach
½-inch piece fresh ginger, peeled
Juice of ½ lemon
¼ cup flat-leaf parsley (optional)

Place all of the ingredients in a blender in the order listed and blend for about 1 minute. Add additional liquid as needed to help with blending.

Place a fine mesh sieve or metal coffee filter over a large bowl. Place pureed beet mixture in sieve and press down with a rubber spatula to extract as much juice as possible. If necessary, strain the beet puree in batches. Chill until ready to drink or serve immediately over ice for a cold drink. Extra juice can be chilled for up to 3 days.

GAME CHANGERS   Use apple juice, cherry juice, or pomegranate juice instead of water ✦ Blend in beet greens or collard greens instead of spinach ✦ Swap out apples in favor of pears ✦ Try lime juice instead of lemon

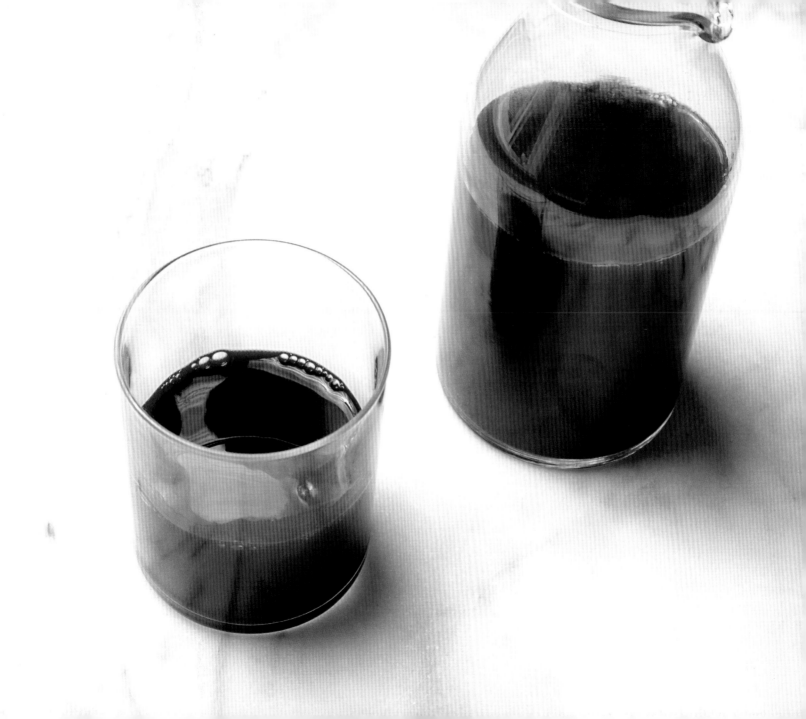

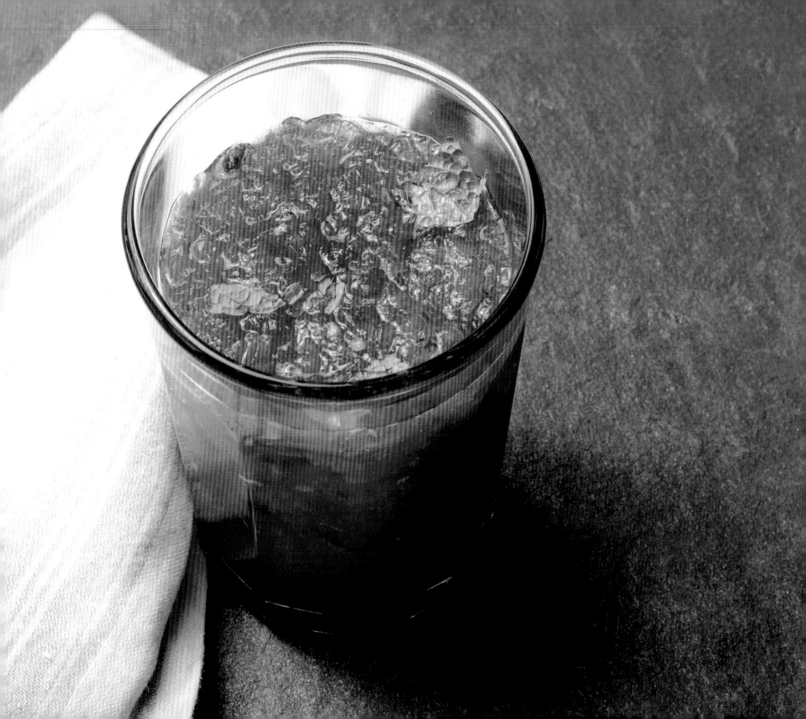

WATERMELON SLUSHY

Rightfully so, watermelon is one of summer's quintessential fruits. And turning it into a heat-busting slushy can ramp up your exercise. Research shows that consuming a frosty slushy before working out in the heat can prolong exercise time. This benefit is likely owing to the ability of the cold drink to reduce core body temperature, which makes exercise seem easier. What's more, a compound called citrulline found in watermelon may help speed up your recovery time by reducing training-induced muscle soreness. So go beyond the wedge.

D G P V

SERVINGS: 1
ACTIVE TIME: 5 min.

You can make a larger batch of the slushy and chill leftovers. When ready for another thirst quencher, simply blend the prepared mixture with additional ice. For transport, pour the prepared slushy into a beverage thermos.

⅓ cup water or coconut water
Juice of ½ lime
1½ cups ice cubes
2 cups cubed seedless watermelon
1 teaspoon honey
1 tablespoon chopped fresh mint (optional)
2 teaspoons chia seeds (optional)

Combine all of the ingredients and a pinch of salt in a blender, and process until you have a slushy consistency. Use the ice-crushing setting on your blender if it has one. Don't overblend into a smooth liquid. Pour into a glass to serve.

GAME CHANGERS Try lemon juice in lieu of lime
+ Use agave syrup instead of honey + Replace mint with basil

MATÉ GINGER ELIXIR

On a recent cycling trip to Argentina, people were carrying thermoses of hot water and gourds stuffed with yerba maté. It turned out the brew offered a much-needed pre-ride buzz on mornings when my legs were tired. Gleaned from leaves of a South American shrub, maté brews up a few different stimulants, including caffeine and theobromine (the "happy" chemical in chocolate), all without coffee's jittery side-effects. As a bonus, a British study found that taking yerba maté before exercise can enhance the fat-burning powers of a workout. This nippy version is a great way to bolster hydration and put a little pep in your step before a hot workout. It's also remarkably refreshing to drink on a sultry day, regardless of any planned exercise. The drink can also be heated on the stove top and transferred to a thermos to help warm your bones on winter excursions. Add honey or agave syrup for a sweeter drink.

SERVINGS: 4
ACTIVE TIME: 10 min.

Beyond subduing the grassy flavor of maté, ginger may help ease any nausea brought on by pre-workout jitters.

You can find maté at many health food stores or tea shops. No loose-leaf? Steep 4 to 5 maté tea bags instead.

3 tablespoons loose-leaf yerba mate
2 teaspoons chopped fresh ginger
¼ cup fresh mint leaves
   Juice of ½ lemon

Place maté, ginger, and mint in a large glass container. Add 4 cups hot water (not boiling), cover, and let steep in the refrigerator overnight. Or place cold water in the container and let the mixture "brew" in a hot, sunny location.

Strain mixture to remove solids and stir in lemon juice. Serve over ice cubes. Store in the fridge for up to 1 week.

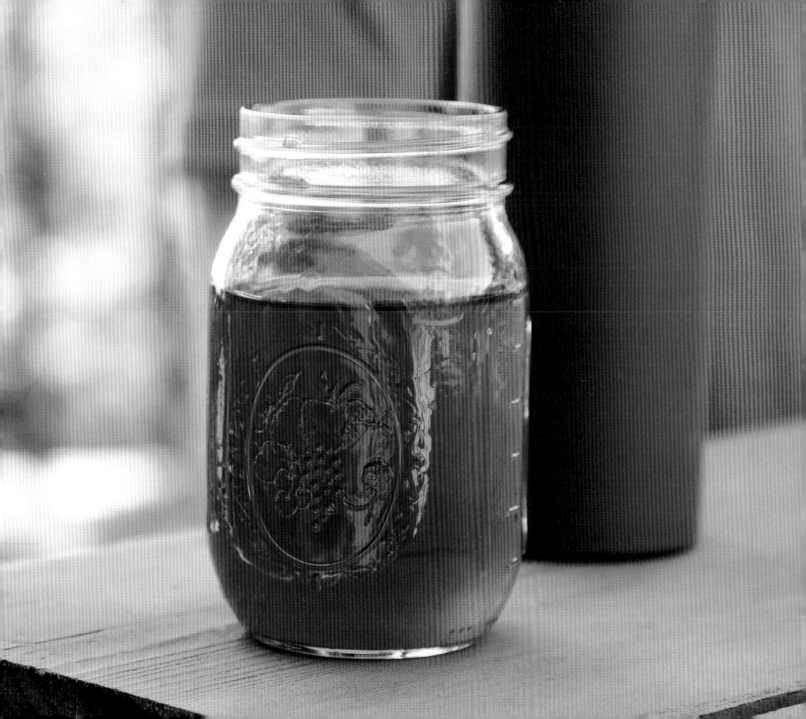

COFFEE CONCENTRATE *(COLD-BREW COFFEE)*

Need an early morning or steamy day pre-workout pick-me-up? Since caffeine can wake up your workout, consider this nitro brew your new best friend. Cold-brewed coffee is simply coffee grounds that are steeped in water without the heat of conventional brewing, resulting in a smoother, less bitter drink. Since this is a concentrate, it's easy to control the strength. Use more coffee and less liquid such as milk for a bigger hit of caffeine, or go the other way for a more mellow drink. For some chocolaty flavor notes, steep 1 tablespoon unsweetened cocoa powder with the coffee grounds.

D G P V

SERVINGS: 6
ACTIVE TIME: 10 min.

When cold water is used to steep coffee grounds, less acid is released, so a glass of cold-brew can be gentler on your digestive system than regular coffee. Also, the longer brewing time and higher grounds-to-water ratio can give the cool brew more of a caffeine jolt per ounce than regular joe. Be cognizant of this if you are prone to the jittery side effects of caffeine before working out.

1 cup coarsely ground coffee beans, preferably a mild or medium roast
1 cinnamon stick, roughly smashed (optional)
4 whole cardamom seeds, gently cracked (optional)
4 cups water

Place ground coffee, cinnamon stick, and cardamom in a large glass container. Add water and stir gently until a light colored foam forms on the surface. Seal shut and let stand at room temperate for 12 to 24 hours.

Use a French press to strain the coffee. Alternatively, pour it through a cheesecloth-lined or coffee filter–lined sieve several times until no grounds appear in the brew, pressing on the solids to remove as much liquid as possible. Store coffee in the refrigerator for up to 1 week.

To serve, place ice in a glass and mix equal amounts of coffee concentrate with water, milk, or a nondairy milk such as almond, hazelnut, or coconut. Try ⅓ to ½ cup of each liquid. Add sweetener of choice, if desired. You can also mix it with some dairy-based or nondairy creamer. Or try one of the alternate recipe options on page 71 to make your brew work harder for you.

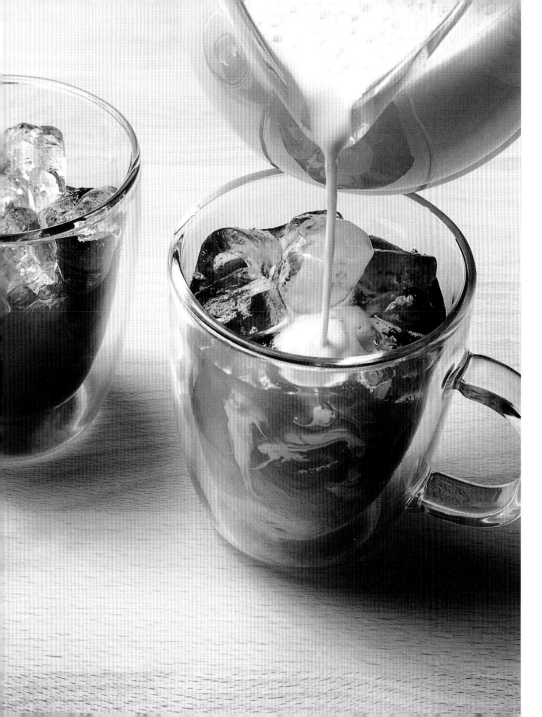

MILKY WAY

Stir together 1 can of evaporated milk and 1 can of sweetened condensed milk. Fill a glass with ice and pour in equal parts coffee concentrate and milk mixture, about ½ cup each.

ENERGY JOLT

To make an exercise energy shot (see p. 137), blend together ⅓ cup coffee concentrate, ¼ cup water, 2 pitted Medjool dates, 1 teaspoon unsweetened cocoa powder, ½ teaspoon vanilla extract, ¼ teaspoon cinnamon, and ⅛ teaspoon salt. Pour into a gel flask.

BERRY MOCHA

To perk up your post-training smoothie, blend together ½ cup coffee concentrate with ½ cup milk, 1 scoop protein powder, 1 tablespoon unsweetened cocoa powder, 2 teaspoons nut or seed butter, 2 teaspoons honey, ½ teaspoon cinnamon, and ½ cup frozen raspberries.

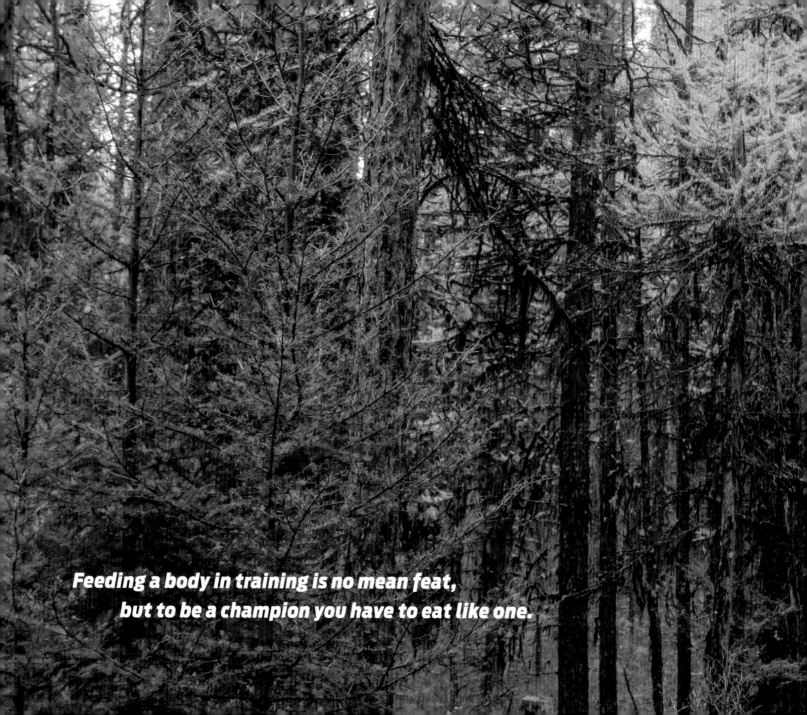

Feeding a body in training is no mean feat,
but to be a champion you have to eat like one.

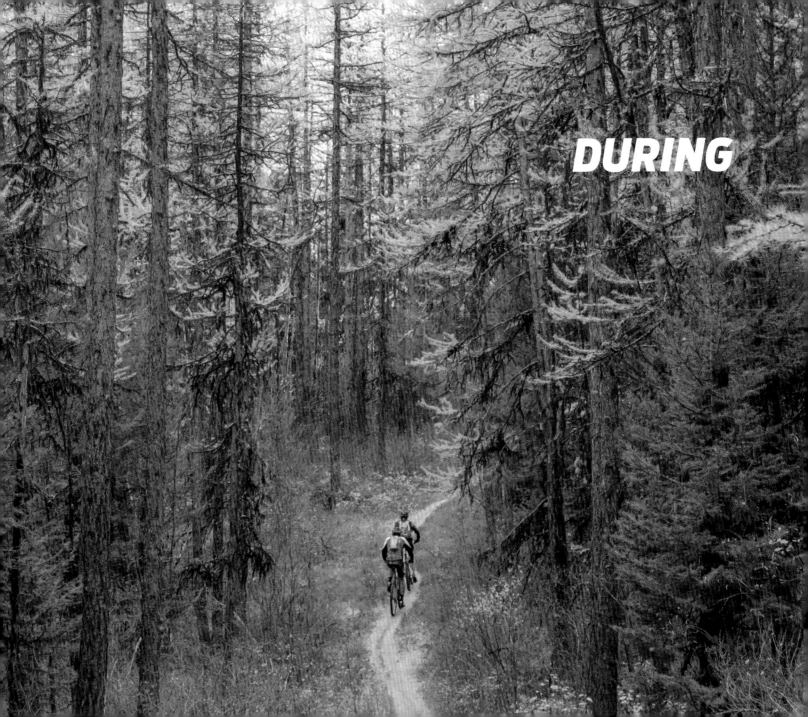

DURING

FUEL THE MACHINE

HITTING THE WALL, bonking, crash and burn. Whatever you call it, it's never fun to experience the unmistakable feeling that your legs are moving through molasses and your brain is full of fog. Having your gas tank hit red is a miserable experience that befalls all levels of athletes at one point or another.

In New Zealand, during my first ride of my very first cycle touring experience, I let myself get way, *way* too low on fuel as I battled a series of spiteful inclines. I ended up staggering into the campground with just enough energy left to spread myself out on a picnic table. I woke up about an hour later with a number of fellow campers peering my way and wondering who this pitiful-looking, sunburnt Canadian was. I now know how to spot the signs of an impending bonk, such as an inability to comprehend a map, and to feast ASAP before reaching the breaking point.

So what exactly causes you to feel completely knackered during exercise, no longer able to keep up the pace or recall what state you are racing in? Most often it's a matter of your body and your brain simply running out of fuel. If you watch nearly any Ironman or ultrarunning event, you'll most likely see a few athletes staggering to the finish line appearing dazed and confused. These are individuals whose muscles and brain are starving for fuel—namely carbohydrates—that is no longer available. The limiting factor for most athletes with highly trained muscles tends to be the availability of energy rather than muscular fatigue.

So to make sure you aren't on the road to a bonk-inducing workout, it's important to recognize the need to provide your body with supplemental energy. Keeping energized during exercise by taking in an appropriate number of calories enables you to push harder and farther so you can fly up the inclines, bust out a few extra reps, and hike up to that postcard-worthy vista you're after. But beyond increasing the amount of time your body can move with gusto, feeding yourself during exercise can help you sidestep a couple other potential problems.

Under-eating during exercise can leave you ravenous upon the cessation of your workout and ready to eat anything and everything in your fridge and pantry. It's an outcome that can derail your training diet. I once staggered into a cheese factory on the Oregon coast after riding too long on too little fuel and ended up eating my body weight in cheddar and Havarti samples. Not only were the employees

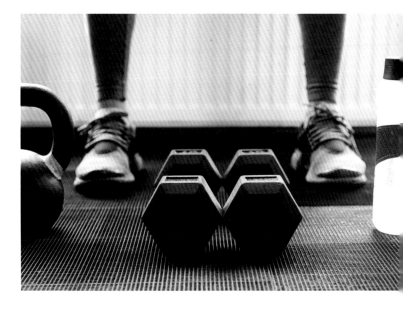

contemplating putting me on their "do not let back in the store" list, but my gut also paid the price from this fat overload.

Also, when you under-eat during a century ride or a full day running the trail, your energy reserves, such as muscle glycogen, can dip so low that it can be a real challenge to try to build them back up to optimal levels. After all, there is only so much pasta you can shovel in after a workout. This is particularly concerning if you have another hard training session or race the following day.

While properly fueling your activity can mean the difference between a brag-worthy performance and one that leaves you crying for mercy and begging for a handful of M&Ms, to reap the full rewards of eating to win it's important to understand when and how to fuel your pursuits.

WATCH THE CLOCK

Not all workouts require you to carbo-load like Chris Froome or Meb Keflezighi. The need for fuel depends greatly on how long and hard you are moving. For the most part, if you are exercising for an hour or less, or even at a moderate pace at the gym for a couple hours (is that you gliding on the elliptical machine while watching *SportsCenter*?), your body likely doesn't require supplemental energy from food beyond a pre-workout snack. Many people overestimate the calories they burn during general workouts, which can easily lead to the consumption of unnecessary calories by guzzling a sports drink or tearing open an energy bar. If you fall into this category, you will get more benefit from perusing the post-workout chapter for some recovery nutrition or using various recipes in this chapter as snack options during the day instead of fuel options during a workout. Assuming that you are consuming a well-balanced diet that contains

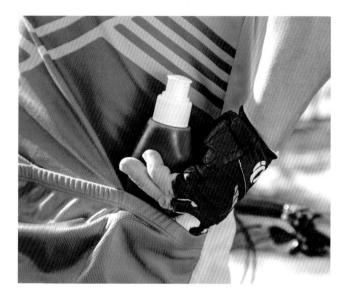

adequate amounts of calories and carbohydrates, you should have sufficient muscle energy reserves to carry you through a workout of this length.

There can be some exceptions to this rule, however. Data is available to suggest that calorie ingestion, primarily in the form of carbs, during shorter bouts of high-intensity exercise (greater than 75 percent of max effort) lasting only 45 to 60 minutes can also give you wings. The going theory is that since your carbohydrate stores are unlikely to be significantly drained during this time frame to the point where you begin feeling sluggish, the performance-boosting benefit likely stems from the stimulation of your central nervous system. So if you're undertaking intense intervals or a stomach-churning CrossFit suffer-fest, you may want to experiment with taking in some fuel, about 30 grams of easily digested carbs, at about the half-hour mark and see if it puts more zip in your step.

The 60- to 90-minute time frame is a gray area when it comes to fueling. Some people can keep on revving along during this time without the need to eat, while others definitely will notice an improvement in performance with some caloric energy during a vigorous workout that goes beyond the hour mark. Just keep in mind that the higher the intensity of exercise, the greater the use of your body's carbohydrate fuel—and the greater the likelihood of extending time to exhaustion with some supplemental fuel increases.

If you're working out hard for 90-plus minutes, you'll likely perform better if you don't leave your homemade bars behind. Eating during these long workouts can help ensure that you don't call it quits early because your blood sugar has taken a nosedive and your energy reserves have been drained. Temperature can also play a role here: The hotter it is, the quicker your body will deplete your glycogen stores, making it necessary for more calories to be consumed.

EMBRACE CARBS

Ready to crush some hills all day long? Well, willpower alone likely won't get you there. There is good reason why athletes know that carbohydrates are the not-so-secret sauce that will keep their workouts moving along. That's because when you train hard, at or above 70 percent of your VO_2max (a measure of the peak amount of oxygen your body can take in and use in a given time), carbs—whether those floating around in your blood as glucose or what is stored in your muscles and liver as glycogen—are your body's preferred fuel. As the intensity increases, so does the percentage of energy used for muscular contraction that will hail from carbs. (At 80 percent of your max effort, up to 90 percent of energy is ideally derived from carbs.) Compared to fat and protein, carbohydrates are very efficient at producing clean energy during intense exercise. So when blood sugar levels fall and glycogen stores become depleted, it becomes a nearly Sisyphean effort to keep going hard and get across the finish line. An evolutionary glitch dictates that our muscle and liver glycogen stores are finite and, in turn, prone to becoming depleted fairly quickly when exercise ramps up. Even those who consume an overall high-carb diet may have only enough glycogen in storage to sustain a couple of hours of vigorous exercise. If you follow a low-carb diet, the clock will begin ticking quicker. So delaying this depletion is critical if you want to maintain intense exercise for a prolonged period of time instead of sputtering along on fumes.

FOR 90+ MIN. OF EXERCISE, TAKE IN 30–90 GRAMS OF CARBS PER HOUR

With low energy reserves, the perception of effort also increases. In other words, you perceive that you're working at a high level, but in actuality your workout output is decreasing—not exactly conducive to nailing that PR.

Also, when your brain senses it is being deprived of carbs, it flips into self-protective mode and restricts the amount available to your working muscles, which can cause your workout to plummet. About 90 percent of your brain's energy comes from carbs, so it has to make sure that it gets what it needs. If not? The quintessential brain fog associated with bonking can set in, and suddenly you can no longer pick good lines on the white water or mountain bike trails.

Consequently, endurance performance and endurance capacity during prolonged activity are largely dictated by external carbohydrate availability in the form of foods and drinks. The mechanisms responsible for the performance benefits of supplemental carbs are related to the prevention of hypoglycemia (drop in blood sugar), the sparing of muscle and liver glycogen, and the allowance for higher rates of carbohydrate-burning for energy production. Research that found that volunteers who swished a carbohydrate-containing drink in their mouths and then spit it out experienced improved performance also suggests there is a central nervous system benefit that is unrelated to the sparing of energy reserves.

Carbohydrate ingestion during exercise has also been shown to be beneficial for individuals participating in sports such as soccer, tennis, and rugby that involve bursts of high-intensity movement. The performance-boosting powers include increased energy and better shooting accuracy with the intake of carbs—roughly 30 to 60 grams for each hour of sport play—and are particularly prevalent during the latter parts of a game, when fatigue often sets in.

GET WHAT YOU NEED

As discussed, if you are dedicated to keeping your workout from moving in slow motion, going without carbohydrates might be the last thing you want to do. For exercise sessions lasting 90-plus minutes you want to shoot for anywhere between 30 and 90 grams of carbohydrates per hour of activity to avoid coming to a standstill. Each gram of carbohydrate delivers 4 calories, giving you 120 to 360 calories during each hour of a workout.

Interestingly, a 2015 study in the *International Journal of Sports Nutrition and Exercise Metabolism* found that trained cyclists who were provided with 39 or 64 grams of carbs in the form of a carbohydrate beverage during each hour of a 2-hour ride performed nearly equally well during a time trial test following the 2-hour ride. Performance suffered, however, when 0 or 20 grams of carbs were administered for each hour of activity. So these results suggest that if your gut doesn't tolerate high intakes of carbs (60 grams or more each hour), you may very well still experience noticeable performance benefits if you take in a little less.

Although this study shows that you may not need to overdose on chews and gels to get enough carbohydrates to power your workout, the precise amount needed will inevitably vary based on a number of factors, including individual tolerance, exercise intensity, exercise duration, one's own metabolism, and environmental conditions. As with pre-exercise nutrition, it's important to experiment during training to determine what works best for you. The best guideline, however, is to look often at your

DO YOU REALLY NEED TO EAT DURING YOUR WORKOUT?

Depending on the type and duration of your workout, you might only need to think about the **BEFORE** and **AFTER** time frames for your fueling needs. For light to moderate workouts lasting an hour or less, most people can get the energy they need from their normal diet, with no extra calories needed during exercise.

	SHORT DURATION	LONG DURATION
LOW INTENSITY	<60 min. workout or light/moderate workout: No fueling necessary	60–90 min. workout: Gauge in training if you benefit from extra fuel
HIGH INTENSITY	45–60 min. workout: Some fuel may help	>90 min. workout: Definitely fuel throughout

specific situation. Going hard all day in the heat? Then you may need to inhale the upper end of the recommended carbohydrate range—up to 90 grams for each hour of activity. Many athletes find that breaking their carbohydrate intake into smaller amounts, say 30 grams every 30 minutes, is easier on their digestive

ELECTRO POWER

Beyond fluid intake, it's imperative that you aim to replace some of the sodium lost during exercise. Beads of sweat aren't just water. In those little drops you'll find a mixture of electrolytes—charged ions necessary to help maintain proper fluid balance as well as regulate muscle contraction and relaxation. So when levels drop too low, your performance can suffer.

Electrolytes lost in the highest concentrations through sweat are sodium and chloride, while those lost in lower amounts include potassium, magnesium, and calcium. For the most part, you need only be concerned with replenishing sodium to maintain optimal bodily functioning, unless you are enduring exercise of extreme lengths such as ultrarunning, where losses of the lesser electrolytes can also become a limiting factor in performance and health.

Sodium's role in helping you move at a faster clip played out in a 2015 *Scandinavian Journal of Medicine and Science in Sports* study that found athletes who supplemented with salt (sodium chloride) in addition to consuming a sports drink before and during a half-Ironman improved race times by an average of 26 minutes compared to those who took a placebo. The performance boost came mostly during the latter parts of the race when electrolyte levels can plummet. The salt supplementation also worked to stimulate thirst, which encouraged subjects to drink more and, in turn, maintain better hydration.

If you're out for a leisurely workout lasting less than an hour, sodium and electrolyte stores should be adequate to carry you through. But replacing salt losses can become necessary when pushing past the 60-minute mark, particularly if you sweat a lot.

Sweat production (and therefore electrolyte loss) is influenced by a number of factors, including humidity, exercise duration and intensity, and genetics. Genetically, some people are salty sweaters, meaning the sodium concentration of their sweat is higher than average. Also, less-fit athletes lose more electrolytes compared to ultra-fit professionals, who are better at maintaining electrolyte balance. Generally, most people lose 300 to 1,000 milligrams of sodium per hour of activity, or between 500 and 1,200 milligrams of sodium in each liter of sweat. Play around with consuming a sodium amount that falls into these ranges during training sessions to pinpoint what works for you. It's not necessary, however, to replace 100 percent of your electrolyte losses—50 to 75 percent should suffice to prevent performance drops. Considering that the typical sports drink contains 200 milligrams or less of sodium, you can see where the need for extra via electrolyte tablets and food from your kitchen can come into play.

system than trying to wolf down an hour's worth of carbs at once, which is not ideal during the latter parts of a workout when you may need to kick it up a notch, making fueling more challenging.

It's also not necessary to try to replace all of the carbs and overall calories that you burn during exercise to still be able to keep up the pace. It can be nearly impossible to consume enough calories to keep up with the amount being burned for energy generation (in some cases 1,000 to 1,500 calories per hour of activity, depending on circumstances such as body weight and intensity) and still maintain good gut function. In general, if you replace about half of the calories you burn during each hour of activity and also start your high-intensity exercise with saturated muscle and liver glycogen stores, you'll be well on your way to a lasting performance.

Although some people will argue that they can function well while taking in fewer carbs than recommended, this often needs to be put into perspective. Functioning and performing optimally may not be one and the same. Lower carbohydrate intake may work if you are exercising for a prolonged time at a constant, low intensity—when a higher percentage of energy is being derived from fat—so there is less pressure on your carbohydrate reserves.

However, performance will likely suffer if you restrict your carb intake during long exercise sessions when the pace is consistently elevated, since at higher intensities, say above 70 to 75 percent of your max effort, human muscles prefer to burn up carbs for energy production. So if you don't continually add some more fuel to your gas tank, your engine won't be able to fire on all cylinders. Still, some athletes are more efficient in that they can perform more work with less fuel. In my case, I seem to not get very great gas mileage and need to refuel regularly to keep going strong.

AT 70–75% MAX EFFORT, YOUR BODY PREFERS CARBS

Many athletes such as Tour de France cyclists will turn to solid foods such as energy bars and homemade goodies for their carb fix during the earlier parts of exercise and then rely more heavily on sources of simple carbohydrates such as sports drinks and gels during the latter parts of an event. As the pace picks up toward the end of a race, the need for fast-digesting carbohydrates to meet energy needs in order to prevent the dreaded bonk becomes more pressing. But if you are really smashing into the wall, you should stop, eat some carbohydrates, and recover before continuing on with exercise.

THINK BEYOND CARBS

Despite me rhapsodizing about carbs, you need not be a slave to them. As long as you are meeting your overall carbohydrate needs, some protein and fat can be a part of your exercise fueling strategy.

Even very lean athletes have enough energy-dense fat stores to fuel hours of walking in the mall or low-intensity exercise (aka the fat-burning zone). A modicum of protein is used for energy-generation purposes, except under extreme workout conditions, when your body can start chomping away at muscles to generate energy. Of interest, the more fit you become, the more you can turn to fat as a fuel source at any given exercise intensity, allowing precious glycogen to be increasingly spared. So while fat and protein are generally not limiting factors to endurance levels in the same way that carbs are, on all-day treks and paddles, protein and fat can deliver a slow stream of energy to help meet overall calorie needs and fend off performance-sapping hunger pangs.

Both of these macronutrients can slow down digestion, but if you are taking part in aerobic exercise for a number of hours, there can be ample time for digestion to take place. So eventually you'll have access to the energy, including that from carbs, found within the protein- or fat-containing foods. This is particularly true if you are working in your fat-burning threshold where the need for carbohydrate consumption is less pressing and blood flow to your gut will likely be higher to aid digestion. Mountaineers, who often work at a steady pace for hours on end, have been known to turn to sticks of butter and pepperoni for their high-altitude nutrition.

Downing only sugary drinks and chews hour after hour is also a recipe for a serious case of gastric distress, otherwise unaffectionately known as "gut rot." I once made the mistake of trying to cram in only high-carbohydrate engineered "race food" during a 24-hour solo mountain biking event. By 2 a.m. my stomach was in a foul mood and I was desperately seeking a slice of cold pizza. One cause of the bloating and gas associated with gut rot is that while exercising, particularly at higher intensities, blood is diverted away from your gut and toward the muscles under stress. This can result in an excess of sugars sitting in your digestive tract for long periods. There, they can begin to ferment in the presence of naturally occurring bacteria.

Snacks that contain some protein and fat also have improved flavor, which functions to stimulate appetite, which can begin to wane as exercise progresses. So helping to relieve palate fatigue by adding moder-

CRAMPING YOUR STYLE

Bananas can be great at giving you the carb fuel needed to torch some serious calories, but the monkey food won't likely keep the cramp monster at bay. Potassium's role in staving off cramps has largely been overblown. You see, cramps are most likely caused when muscles such as those in the calf become overstressed during prolonged, intense exercise or from inadequately training your muscles to handle the situation at hand. Think about when you last had a neck or bicep cramp during a long run. Um, never! Although neuron misfiring in response to muscles under pressure is the main culprit of cramping, significant dehydration or an electrolyte imbalance, particularly excessive salt loss, can also play a role.

ate amounts of fat and protein can encourage an athlete to keep on eating and meeting caloric needs.

Bodybuilders have long consumed some protein, mostly in the form of amino acids blended with water or a sports drink, as a means to stymie some of the muscle breakdown that can occur during a workout. Indeed, a bit of protein in your exercise fuel can serve to help preserve muscle during bouts of intense resistance training or when you are moving

for several hours, such as during a backpacking trip or a marathon mountain bike race, which is ideal for overall fitness.

Because everyone responds differently to the fuel they eat, I want to once again stress the importance of experimenting during training periods with a variety of foods and drinks with various macronutrient composition. Don't be afraid to try items that buck the trends of sports nutrition marketing—think Blini Sliders (p. 127) or Hand Pies (p. 128) instead of packaged bars. If possible, try to use foods and drinks at the same rates as you would in a race. Listening to your gut is often a better idea than listening to the marketing hype. Stay committed to what you know works best for you.

LIQUID ASSETS

On top of taking in sufficient carbs and overall calories, maintaining sound hydration habits during exercise results in better performance. As little as 2 to 3 percent body-weight loss caused by dehydration can impair performance via a loss in power and speed during a prolonged workout, even if you have sufficient energy reserves remaining. If it feels like you are running through Jell-O halfway through a workout, perhaps it's dehydration that is slowing you down. Beyond a 5 percent loss in body weight, the risk of heat-related illnesses such as heatstroke is greatly heightened. Dehydration can tame your exercise by increasing core temperature, reducing blood flow, and accelerating muscle glycogen use. Adequate fluid is also necessary for the proper absorption of the nutrients found in your fuel of choice. When hydration is available in subpar amounts, digestion can slow down, leading to gastrointestinal problems and reduced availability of fuel for your working muscles.

DRINK
400–1,000 MILLILITERS
OF FLUID
EACH HOUR
OF EXERCISE

To sidestep dehydration, aim to chug back 400 to 1,000 milliliters of fluid each hour of exercise by sipping smaller amounts frequently every 20 minutes or so. Your precise fluid needs will be dictated by a number of factors, including your individual sweat rate, the temperature at which exercise is taking place, and the intensity of activity. During a hot, intense workout, you'll want to shoot for the higher end of this fluid-intake range. Your fluid needs can be met by using a sports drink, water spiked with an electrolyte tablet, or even plain tap water as long as you are also considering your overall need for carbohydrates and electrolytes from other sources. Real foods such as fruit and rice also supply some fluid to the active body.

A good way to ensure that you are drinking enough fluid during training and races is to weigh yourself before and after exercise to obtain a better grasp of how factors such as intensity or ambient temperature impact your fluid needs. For the most part, the weight shed during activity is water weight, with a very small amount being burnt-up energy reserves. Ideally, you want to make it a goal not to finish a workout with a 3 percent or greater drop in body weight. If you do lose that much, try to drink a little more during your next outing. Not needing to take any nature breaks during several hours of activity is also an indication that you're not meeting your fluid needs. You can work toward replacing each lost pound of body weight by consuming 2 to 3 cups of liquid post-workout.

On the flip side, you don't want to overhydrate to the point of developing hyponatremia, a potentially fatal condition where you are essentially diluting your sodium to dangerously low levels. When the concentration of sodium in the fluids surrounding cells in the body drops as a result of drinking too much sodium-free fluid, water moves into the cells to balance things out. This unfortunately causes cells to swell, including those found in the brain, which can lead to confusion,

KEEP
WEIGHT LOST
DURING
EXERCISE TO
3 PERCENT
OR LESS

headaches, and even death in extreme cases. To limit the risk for hyponatremia, consume fluids or foods that contain sodium during prolonged sweat-inducing exercise but don't overdose on fluid to the point where you finish a workout actually weighing more than you did to begin with. Think of your weekend warrior who is out running in a multi-hour marathon or spending the day in the saddle during a Gran Fondo and drinking too much water without much thought about sodium or sweat rates. A *British Journal of Sports Medicine* study reviewed previously published data and found enough evidence to suggest that drinking when thirsty during exercise can be enough to allow an active person to maintain proper hydration.

GET IN THE KITCHEN

When it comes to fueling your body, there are now endless choices on store shelves. But if you spend a lot of time on the trail or in the saddle, choking down copious amounts of packaged gels and bars can get old. That's why more and more athletes are spending more time in the kitchen making up batches of their own endurance fuel, which can provide the necessary nutrition in a healthier, better-tasting form.

In addition to the taste difference, science is increasingly finding that wholesome foods without the sci-fi–sounding ingredients can work just as well as prepackaged products to bolster your workouts. For example, researchers from the University of California, Davis, tuckered out participants by having them run for 80 minutes and then complete a 5K time trail while consuming either water, water and carb-rich chews, or water and raisins. The end result was that when runners consumed the raisins or sports chews, they ran their 5K on average one minute faster than when they ingested only water. Most important, there was no difference in performance between the chews and the much less-expensive raisin trials. This result strongly suggests that the sugars in the shriveled grapes were efficiently burned up for energy production.

More proof that natural energy works: Researchers at Appalachian State University, North Carolina, had cyclists either drink a cup of a 6 percent carbohydrate sports drink or eat half a banana and a cup of water every 15 minutes during a 46-mile pedal. In the end, both groups finished in the same amount of time. Similarly, a *Journal of Strength and Conditioning Research* study found that honey was just as effective as dextrose, which is a form of glucose, at boosting endurance. Research suggests consuming items such as honey and dried fruit, which contain a blend of sugars such as fructose and glucose, during exercise

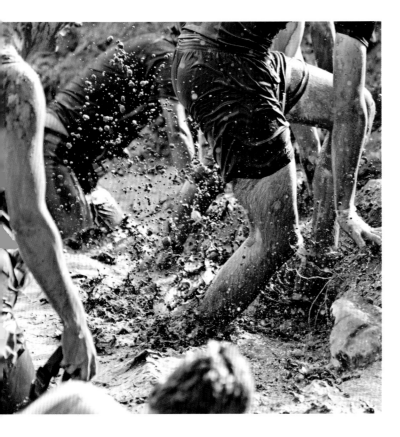

can be particularly effective at increasing the digestive rate, and in turn the burning rate, of carbs.

Another benefit of fueling during extended exercise with real-food items is that it's an opportunity to provide your active body with more of the nutrients it needs to be healthy and perform optimally. Athletes should think beyond breakfast, lunch, and dinner as a means to meeting their overall nutritional needs.

With all of that in mind, I have increasingly been relying on real foods like the DIY bars, energy shots, and wraps that populate the following recipes to fuel my activities. I still do sometimes turn to store-bought items, including chews and gels, but I'm cognizant of the benefits of pairing these with sweet and savory stuff from my kitchen. My mood on the bike always seems better if I've got some Brownie Bites (p. 125) or Millet Cherry Bars (p. 102) within arm's reach. If you are someone who needs quite a bit of supplemental energy during prolonged exercise, I think you'll find that homemade fuel options encourage you to eat more.

If you're like me and the thought of another packaged gel is hard to stomach, the recipes that follow will deliver all of these nutritional benefits in tasty, transportable packages of energy that serve to wake up your palate. After all, food is meant to be enjoyable. Keep in mind that some recipes, like the unique Trail Mix options (p. 90), are designed more for outings that allow for pack space and snack breaks, such as backpacking or paddling, as they don't necessarily make a great option for stuffing into your jersey pocket. But other fuel creations, such as the

Energy Shots (p. 137) and Enduro Balls (p. 110), can be brought along on a long ride, run, or climb to help power you through to the end—minus the dreaded gut rot. Or, turn your next group ride or run into an on-the-go potluck by having everyone make a recipe to share. There are endless ways to savor the miles you spend on the road or the trail.

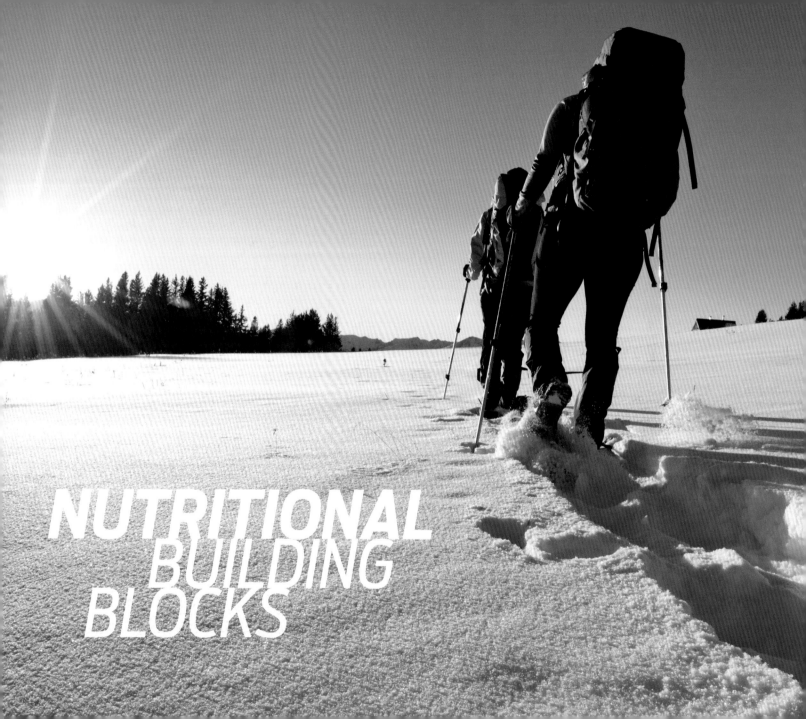

NUTRITIONAL
BUILDING
BLOCKS

RECIPES FOR **DURING**

D Dairy-free   F Freezer-friendly   G Gluten-free   P Paleo-friendly   V Vegetarian or vegan-friendly

Look to the Game Changers section to find simple substitutions that make nearly every recipe more friendly for specific diets.

TRAIL MIX

Whether backpacking, canoeing, or car camping, trailblazers have long known that a stash of energy-dense trail mix can power any exploration. The following gussied-up versions prove that time-honored trail mix can be so much more than peanuts and raisins. With these trail mixes on hand, you'll be happy to go out and embrace the outdoors.

D G V

SERVINGS: 8
ACTIVE TIME: 10 min.

Bulk bins are a great place to locate items such as dried fruit and nuts in just the right portions you need for making trail mix.

GOURMET PIZZA

2–3 ounces herb crackers, broken into ½-inch pieces*

2–3 ounces pepperoni or other cured meat such as jerky, chopped

2 ounces feta cheese, crumbled (about ½ cup)

½ cup unsalted roasted almonds

½ cup sliced dried figs

½ cup thinly sliced sun-dried tomatoes (not oil packed)

¼ cup raw shelled pumpkin seeds (pepitas)

* Add crackers no more than 2 days before serving to keep them crisp.

TROPICAL TWISTER

4 cups plain popcorn

½ cup chopped dried mango

½ cup chopped dried pineapple

½ cup unsalted shelled pistachios

½ cup roughly chopped unsalted dry-roasted cashews

⅓ cup unsweetened flaked coconut

¼ cup wasabi peas

2 nori sheets, torn into small pieces

CHERRY HAZE

2 cups brown rice crisps or puffs

½ cup halved hazelnuts

½ cup pecans

½ cup dried cherries

½ cup dried blueberries

½ cup dark chocolate chips

⅓ cup unsweetened flaked coconut

¼ cup raw shelled pumpkin seeds (pepitas)

CRUNCHY APPLE

2 ounces sweet potato chips, roughly broken apart (about 1 cup)

1½–2 ounces plain or cinnamon apple chips, roughly broken (about ¾ cup)

1 cup roughly chopped walnuts

¾ cup dried cranberries

⅓ cup raw shelled pumpkin seeds (pepitas)

¼ cup cacao nibs

Place all of the ingredients for each trail mix combination in a large container and toss to combine. Divide mixture among zip-top bags for transport. Mixes can be made up to 3 days in advance.

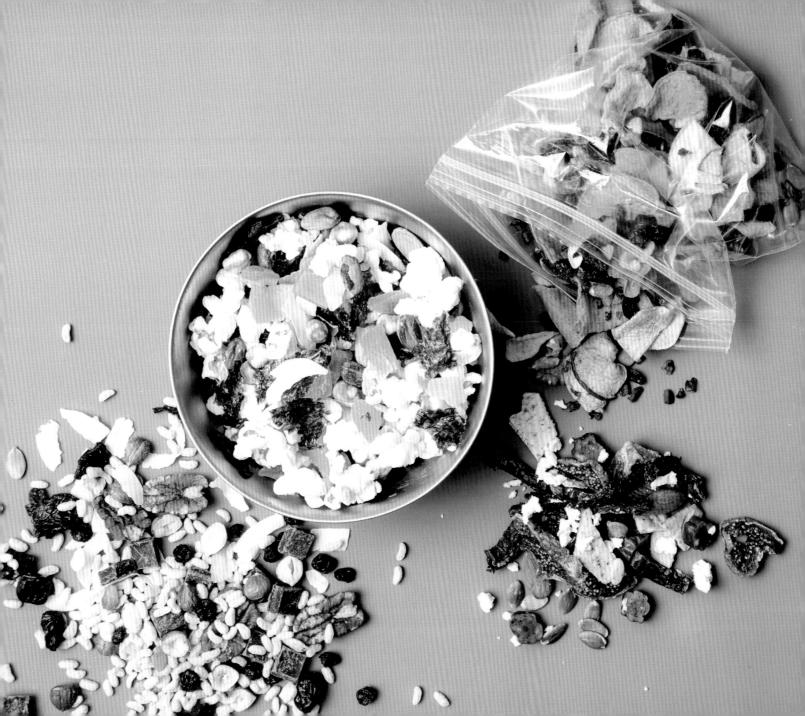

MAPLE BANANA CHIPS

With these oven-dried banana chips there is no need to stuff a whole banana in your jersey pocket or backpack only to find fruit mush when you're famished. They still retain just the right amount of moisture and great banana flavor—nothing like the lackluster chips on offer from the bulk bins. These chips can also be prepared in a food dehydrator.

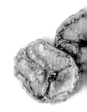

D G P V

SERVINGS: 4
ACTIVE TIME: 15 min.

The best bananas to use for this recipe are ones with a few dark spots on their skin. Overly ripe ones will be too mushy to properly slice, while green on the skin indicates the fruit is not yet at its sweet best.

2 medium-sized bananas
2 tablespoons pure maple syrup
⅛ teaspoon salt

Preheat oven to 200°F. Line a baking sheet with parchment paper and lightly grease.

Thinly slice bananas and place them in a single layer on baking sheet. Brush banana slices with maple syrup and then sprinkle on salt. Bake for 1 hour 40 minutes, or until most of the moisture has been removed from the bananas. Let cool before placing in small zip-top bags for transport, or chill for up to 3 days.

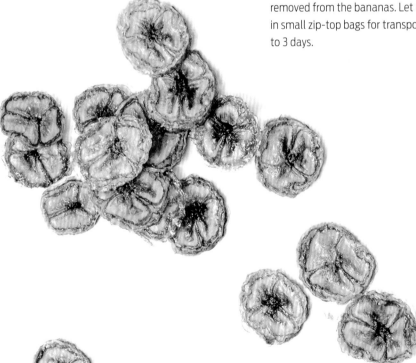

APRICOT BANANA SAMMIES

When your body is starting to run flat, these bundles of fruity energy will put the zip back into your stride or pedal stroke. Cooking the banana down serves to concentrate its flavor. The resulting spreadable chocolate banana butter is also stellar when slathered on Blinis (p. 127).

SERVINGS: 8
ACTIVE TIME: 20 min.

To hasten banana ripening, see the method suggested in the Flourless Protein Banana Muffins recipe (p. 209).

2 medium-sized very ripe bananas
1 tablespoon fresh lemon juice
1 ounce dark chocolate, finely chopped
½ teaspoon vanilla extract
¼ teaspoon cinnamon
32 dried apricots

Place bananas in a medium-sized saucepan and mash with a potato masher or a fork. Stir in lemon juice. Bring to a boil and simmer, uncovered, over medium heat until liquid has been cooked off, about 15 minutes, stirring often. Be careful not to let the banana burn on the bottom of the pan. Remove from heat, stir in chocolate, vanilla, cinnamon, and a pinch of salt until chocolate has melted. Let cool. The finished banana butter can be stored in the fridge for up to 4 days.

To assemble, place a small amount of chocolate banana butter on an apricot half and press on another apricot half. Repeat with the rest of the apricots. Transfer to small zip-top bags for transport.

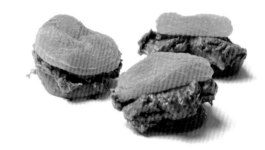

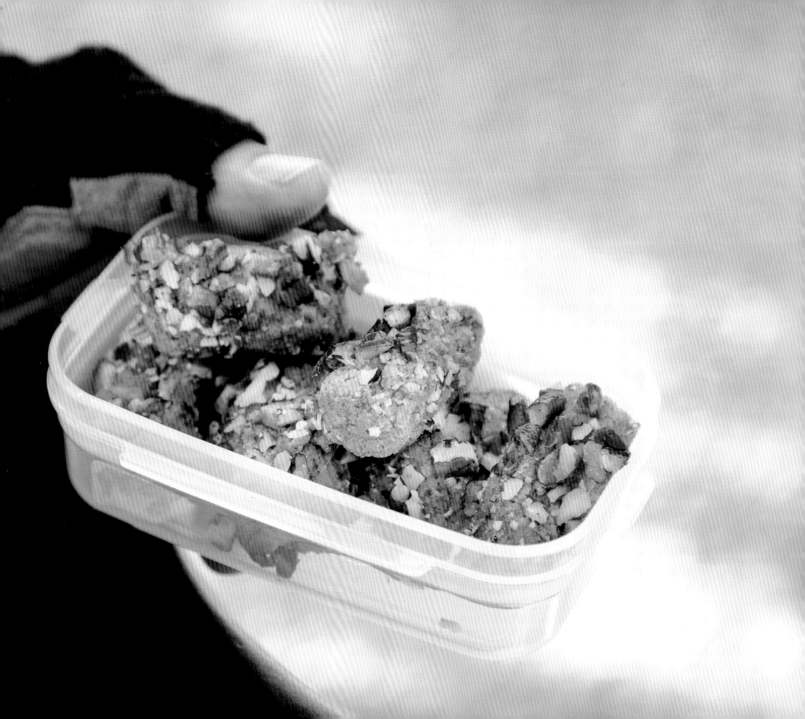

SWEET POTATO TOTS

Tender on the inside with a nutty crisp on the outside, these energy bombs flip a switch that tells your body to move harder, faster, and longer. The secret ingredient is coconut flour, which works its magic to absorb some of the excess moisture from the mashed potato so the tots will firm up and better keep their shape during transport. To make these even more crave-worthy, I'll often mix a couple of tablespoons of molasses into the potato mash.

D G P V

SERVINGS: 12
ACTIVE TIME: 25 min.

To freeze and bake later, place formed tots on a baking sheet and freeze. Once frozen solid, place in an airtight container and store in the freezer until needed. When it's time to fuel your pursuit, place frozen tots on a baking sheet and bake for about 15 to 20 minutes longer than the recipe calls for.

1½ pounds sweet potatoes (about 2 medium-sized), peeled and cubed
¼ cup coconut flour
½ teaspoon cinnamon
¼ teaspoon salt
¾ cup finely chopped pecans
2 tablespoons coconut sugar or brown sugar

Steam or boil sweet potatoes until fork-tender. Place cooked sweet potato in a bowl and mash until smooth. Stir in coconut flour, cinnamon, and salt. In a separate small bowl, stir together pecans and sugar.

Preheat oven to 375°F and line a baking sheet with parchment paper or a silicone baking mat. Scoop out sweet potato mixture by the tablespoon and roll between hands into a cylindrical shape. Roll in pecan mixture and place on baking sheet. Chop more pecans if needed. You should have about 24 tots.

Bake for 40 minutes, flipping halfway, or until golden on the outside. They will firm up further upon cooling. Tots can be kept in the refrigerator for up to 5 days. If you want to enjoy them warm as a snack, simply microwave tots for about 30 seconds.

GAME CHANGERS Season with allspice instead of cinnamon + Use finely chopped walnuts instead of pecans + Substitute date sugar for coconut or brown sugar

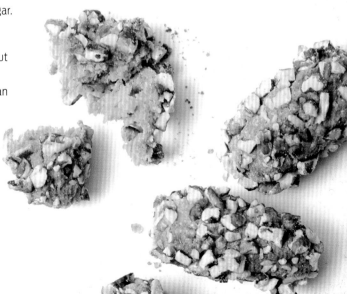

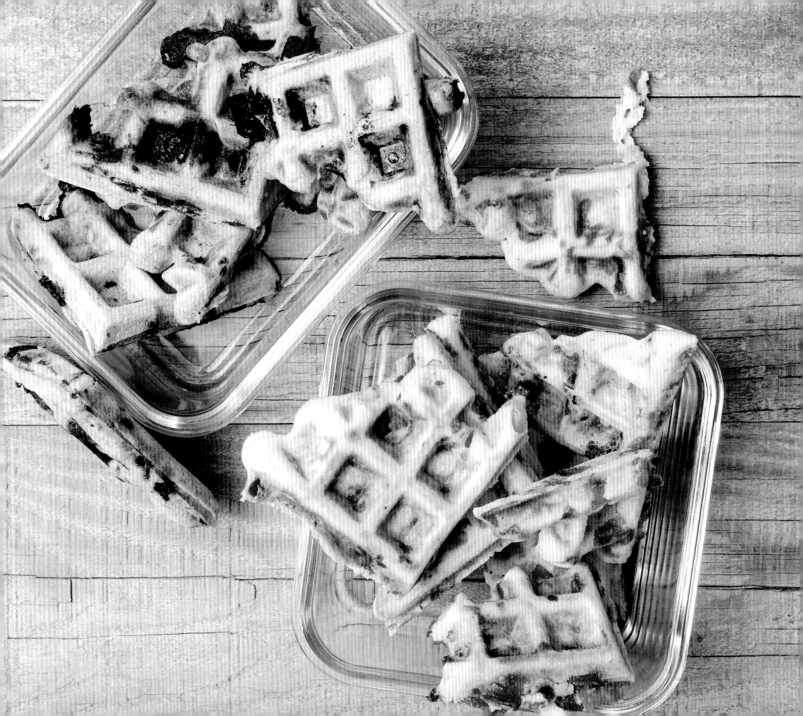

WAFFLE BITES

Time to dust off the waffle iron! Here's proof that waffles shouldn't be pigeonholed for breakfast or brunch. These sweet and savory incarnations are a creative replacement for staid, old energy bars when your weary muscles are begging for nourishment. Exercise never tasted so good.

D F G V

SERVINGS: 8
ACTIVE TIME: 20 min.

The waffle batters can be made up 2 days in advance if kept chilled. Bring up to room temperature before using.

WAFFLE 'ZAS

- 1 cup all-purpose flour or 1-to-1 gluten-free flour blend
- 1 teaspoon baking powder
- 1½ teaspoons dried oregano
- 1 teaspoon onion powder
- 1 large egg, lightly beaten
- 1 cup low-fat milk
- 2 tablespoons olive oil
- 3 ounces shredded reduced-fat mozzarella (about ¾ cup)
- 2 ounces diced pepperoni
- ½ cup diced green bell pepper
- ¼ cup diced oil-packed sun-dried tomatoes

BERRY CHOCOLATE

- 1 cup oat flour or all-purpose flour
- 1 teaspoon baking powder
- 1 teaspoon cinnamon
- ¼ teaspoon salt
- 1 large egg, lightly beaten
- ¾ cup plain almond milk or low-fat milk
- 1 ripe banana, mashed
- ½ cup fresh blueberries
- ⅓ cup dark chocolate chips
- 1 teaspoon lemon zest

In a large bowl, whisk together flour, baking powder, and any dry seasonings. In a separate bowl, whisk together the egg and liquid ingredients. Add wet ingredients to dry ingredients and mix just until everything is moist. If needed, add more milk, a tablespoon at a time, if batter is too thick. Fold in any extras such as cheese or chocolate chips.

Grease a waffle iron with cooking spray and heat according to the manufacturer's instructions. Ladle about ⅔ cup batter for each waffle into waffle iron and heat until golden brown and cooked through. You should get at least 4 waffles. Let cool on a wire rack and then slice each waffle into quarters for transport. Prepared waffles can also be wrapped tightly and frozen for up to 1 month.

HASH BROWN BACON PATTIES

When you are suffering gel and bar fatigue, these portable hash browns are sure to lift your spirits and keep you moving strong. Gleaned from the back of the hog, Canadian-style bacon (peameal bacon in Canuck parlance) is significantly leaner than traditional bacon, so it won't bog you down with excess fat calories.

D F G P

SERVINGS: 8
ACTIVE TIME: 25 min.

You can also try making these all at once by scooping the potato mixture onto a greased or parchment paper–lined baking sheet and baking at 400°F for about 15 minutes per side, or until hash browns are darkened and crispy.

½ pound thinly sliced Canadian-style bacon
1 pound sweet potato (about 1 large), peeled and finely grated
½ cup all-purpose flour
2 large eggs, lightly whisked
2 large egg whites
1 tablespoon fresh thyme
1 teaspoon garlic powder
1 teaspoon onion powder
1 tablespoon canola, grapeseed, or coconut oil

Cook bacon in a lightly oiled skillet over medium-low heat until it begins to brown and turn crispy, about 2 to 3 minutes per side. Transfer to a paper towel–lined cutting board and let cool. Once cool, finely chop bacon.

In a large bowl, combine bacon, shredded potatoes, flour, eggs, egg whites, thyme, garlic powder, and onion powder.

Heat oil in skillet over medium heat. For each patty, scoop about ¼ cup potato mixture into skillet, gently flatten with a spatula or back of a measuring cup, and cook 2 to 3 minutes per side, or until golden and set. Let hash browns cool on metal racks and repeat with remaining potato mixture, adding more oil to skillet as needed. You should end up with roughly 16 patties. Store in refrigerator for up to 5 days, or freeze for up to 1 month.

GAME CHANGERS Use a gluten-free flour such as rice instead of all-purpose flour + Try almond flour for Paleo-friendly hash browns + Mix in chopped rosemary instead of thyme

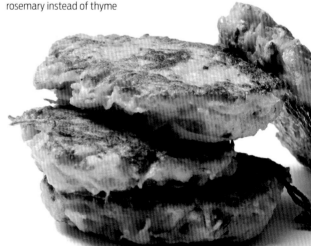

PESTO POTATO PATTIES

A favorite among backcountry campers, dehydrated potato flakes can be transformed into pancake-like patties that deliver the easily digested carbs needed to hit top-end speeds. For a little zing, you can stir some lemon zest into the potato batter.

D F G V

SERVINGS: 5
ACTIVE TIME: 15 min.

For fresher flavor, consider making your own pesto: Place 3 cups arugula, ½ cup basil or mint, ⅓ cup walnuts or ¼ cup hemp seeds, ⅓ cup grated Parmesan cheese, 1 garlic clove, and ¼ teaspoon salt in a food processor and blend until greens are pulverized. With the machine running, pour in ¼ cup extra-virgin olive oil and juice of ½ lemon until incorporated, scraping down the sides as needed.

1½ cups instant potato flakes
2 large eggs, lightly beaten
2–3 tablespoons prepared pesto
⅓ cup finely chopped oil-packed sun-dried tomatoes
1 tablespoon butter or oil

Place potato flakes in a large bowl. Add 1½ cups hot water. Add eggs and stir quickly until batter becomes somewhat thick. Stir in pesto and sun-dried tomatoes.

Heat butter or oil in a skillet over medium heat. Place ¼ cup batter for each patty in skillet and press down gently to flatten. Cook until golden brown on both sides, about 4 minutes per side. Let cool on metal racks and repeat with remaining potato batter. You should end up with about 10 patties. Chill for up to 5 days and transport in a small zip-top bag.

GAME CHANGERS Swap out pesto for chopped herbs such as chives or basil **+** For dairy-free cakes, use pesto made without cheese **+** Use chopped roasted red pepper instead of sun-dried tomatoes

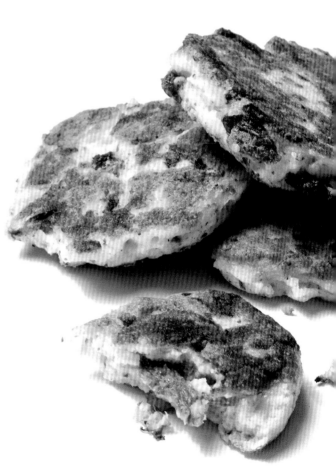

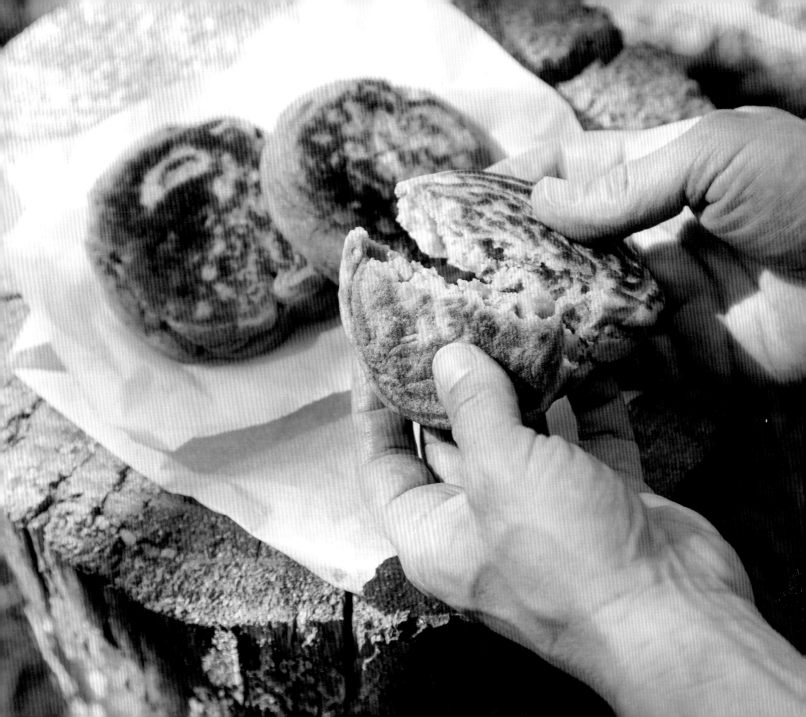

INSIDE-OUT PANCAKES

This whimsical twist on a breakfast classic, with the topping hiding within, is a much more fun way to get your energy-boosting carbs than the standard packaged stuff. These are also perfect for road trips and camping.

SERVINGS: 5
ACTIVE TIME: 25 min.

To quicken the pace, you could also use a store-bought pancake mix.

Cooling these and other items like muffins on metal racks lets air circulate around them, which prevents soggy bottoms.

1 cup all-purpose flour

1 teaspoon cinnamon, divided

1 teaspoon baking powder

¼ teaspoon baking soda

⅛ teaspoon salt

1 large egg, lightly beaten

¾ cup buttermilk or low-fat milk

1 medium-sized pear, finely chopped

1 tablespoon brown sugar or coconut sugar

1 tablespoon fresh lemon juice

In a large bowl, stir together flour, ½ teaspoon cinnamon, baking powder, baking soda, and salt. Stir in egg and buttermilk or milk and mix until smooth. If batter is too thick, stir in additional liquid, 1 tablespoon at a time, until you reach a fairly thin consistency.

In a separate bowl, stir together pear, sugar, lemon juice, and ½ teaspoon cinnamon.

Heat a nonstick skillet, griddle, or cast-iron pan over medium heat. Grease as needed. Place 1 tablespoon batter in pan and top with about 1 tablespoon of the pear mixture. Top with another tablespoon of batter so that pears are covered. Cook until edges begin to darken, flipping after about 2 minutes. Cook 1 minute more. Repeat with remaining batter and pear filling. You should end up with about 10 pancakes. Let pancakes cool on wire racks.

GAME CHANGERS Use 1-to-1 gluten-free flour blend, spelt flour, whole wheat pastry flour, or oat flour instead of all-purpose flour ✦ Replace buttermilk or regular cow milk with nondairy milk such as almond ✦ Fill with chopped apples or peaches instead of pears

MILLET CHERRY BARS

Here's more proof that you don't need to dish out your hard-earned cash for energy bars designed in factories when making your own inspiring version is easy, even for the culinary challenged. Not just for the birds, millet is an inexpensive gluten-free grain that gives these bars great texture and nutritional firepower.

D F G V

SERVINGS: 9
ACTIVE TIME: 20 min.

The flat side of a measuring cup is a perfect tool for pressing the bar mixture into a flat, even layer in the pan. Also, placing the uncut bars in the refrigerator for a couple of hours can make slicing them easier.

1 cup roughly chopped pecans
½ cup raw millet
¼ cup raw shelled sunflower seeds
¼ cup raw shelled pumpkin seeds (pepitas)
1 cup dried cherries
2 tablespoons honey
  Zest of 1 medium orange
½ teaspoon salt

Preheat oven to 350°F. Spread pecans, millet, sunflower seeds, and pumpkin seeds on a rimmed baking sheet. Place in oven and heat, stirring a couple times, until golden and fragrant, 10 to 12 minutes.

Line an 8 × 8–inch square baking pan with a piece of parchment paper large enough so there is a 1-inch overhang.

Reduce oven temperature to 200°F. Blend cherries, honey, orange zest, salt, and 2 tablespoons water in a food processor into a paste. Transfer to a bowl and stir in toasted pecan mixture. Press firmly into prepared pan in an even layer and bake until just slightly sticky to the touch, 25 to 30 minutes. Let cool completely in pan before using the parchment overhang to lift from pan. Cut into 9 bars. These can be kept chilled for 2 weeks or frozen for up to 2 months if wrapped tightly.

GAME CHANGERS Replace pecans with almonds + Try raw quinoa as a replacement for millet + Swap out cherries for cranberries + Use brown rice syrup or agave syrup instead of honey + Add lemon zest instead of orange zest

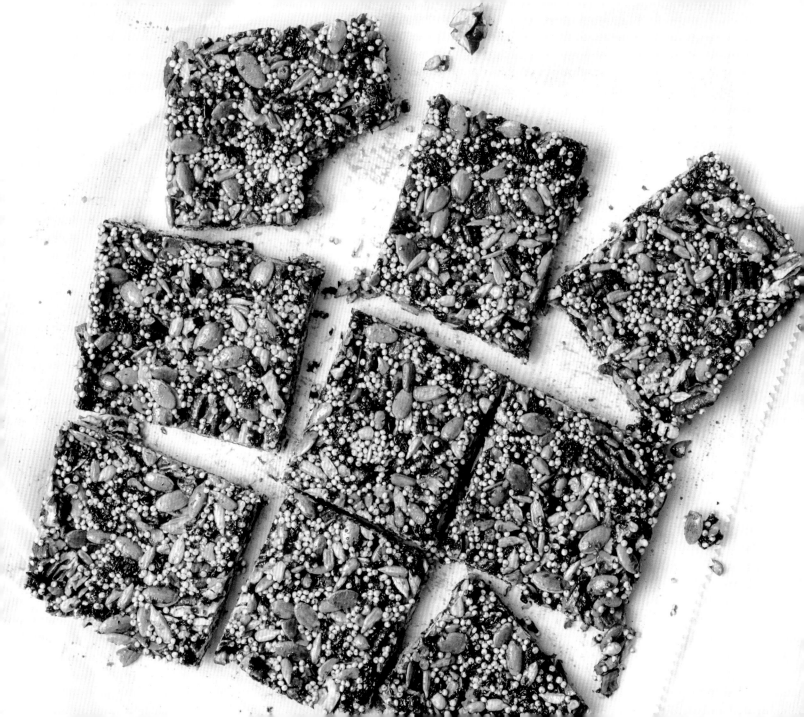

SMOKY HONEY MUSTARD BARS

One of the best things to happen to the oversaturated energy bar market in recent times is the introduction of savory flavors for a change of pace, so I thought I'd create a bar with those flavor hooks in mind. These not only deliver the energy you need, they also make your workout fuel taste reminiscent of a backyard barbecue. They're great as a snack or pre-exercise bite as well.

D F G V

SERVINGS: 9
ACTIVE TIME: 20 min.

Liquid smoke is available in nearly every grocery store by the barbecue sauce. Look for one with only two ingredients: water and smoke—no flavoring agents or colorants. A little goes a long way. Corn syrup is a better binder than honey, but if you want to steer clear of GMO corn, you can opt for an organic brand such as Wholesome Sweeteners.

2 cups puffed rice cereal
⅔ cup roughly chopped raw almonds
⅓ cup raw shelled pumpkin seeds (pepitas)
3 tablespoons hemp seeds
¼ cup honey
3 tablespoons light corn syrup
2 tablespoons almond butter
1 tablespoon yellow mustard powder
1 teaspoon garlic powder
1 teaspoon onion powder
1 teaspoon liquid smoke
½ teaspoon salt
¼ teaspoon black pepper

Combine puffed cereal, almonds, pumpkin seeds, and hemp seeds in a large bowl.

Place honey, corn syrup, and almond butter in a small saucepan. Bring to a simmer and heat until mixture is liquefied. Stir in mustard powder, garlic powder, onion powder, liquid smoke, salt, and black pepper. Add honey mixture to bowl with cereal mixture and stir to combine.

Line an 8 × 8–inch square baking pan with a piece of parchment paper large enough so there is a 1-inch overhang. Place bar mixture in pan and press down firmly into an even layer. Chill in refrigerator for at least 2 hours to set. Carefully lift out of pan with parchment overhang and slice into 9 bars. Store in the refrigerator for up to 10 days. Wrap individual bars tightly in foil or other wrapper of choice for transport.

GAME CHANGERS Use puffed quinoa, wheat, or millet instead of rice + Swap out almonds for pecans + Replace hemp seeds with sunflower seeds + Use peanut butter instead of almond butter

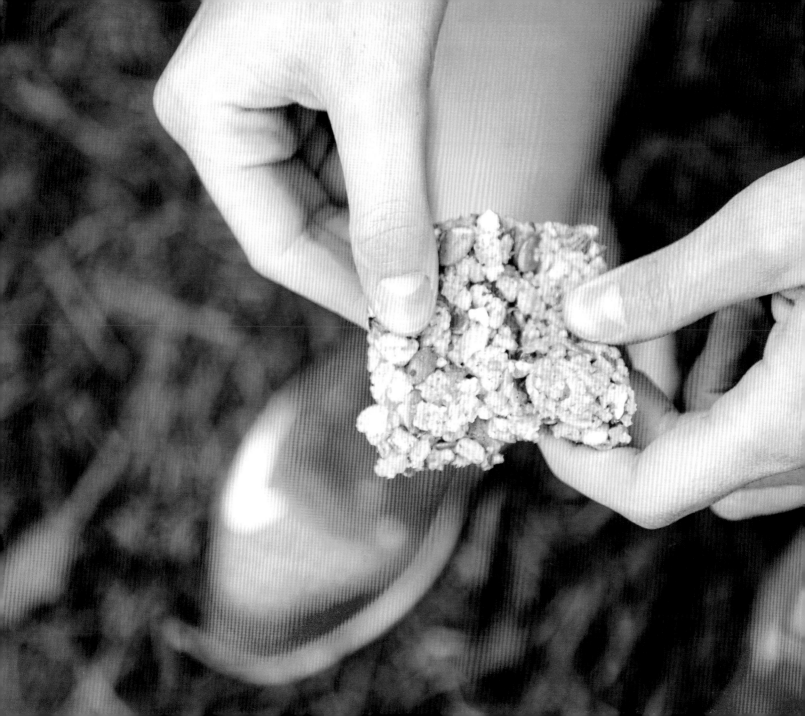

COCONUT RICE CAKES

From the punishing mountains of northern Thailand to the temple-studded plains of Myanmar to the dusty roads of Cambodia, I've come to rely on various forms of coconut-sweetened rice cakes as efficient fuel to energize my rides throughout Asia. The banana leaf–wrapped purple rice cakes with coconut custard from the morning market in Luang Prabang, Laos, are worth the flight alone. This mango-infused version holds together well when you are out and about, and it supplies easily digestible, toothsome energy. And the cooked rice is nearly 70 percent water, adding extra fluid that you won't find in most packaged energy bars.

D F G V

SERVINGS: 12
ACTIVE TIME: 20 min.

Coconut flour is made by grinding up defatted dried coconut meat into a fine powder.

Don't try to cut corners by leaving out the coconut flour. You need it to help draw out some of the excess moisture during baking so that the cakes hold together.

1 cup medium-grain white rice, such as Calrose
½ teaspoon salt
1 cup light coconut milk
1 mango, preferably Altaulfo, peeled and sliced
⅔ cup coconut sugar
3 large eggs
⅓ cup coconut flour
¼ cup sesame seeds (optional)

Rinse rice in a sieve under cold water. Bring 2 cups water to a boil in a medium-sized saucepan. Add rice and salt, stir, and return to a boil. Reduce heat to low and simmer, covered, for 15 minutes, or until rice is tender and water has been absorbed. Remove from heat, let sit covered for 5 minutes, and then fluff with a fork.

Preheat oven to 350°F. Line an 8 × 8–inch square baking pan with a piece of parchment paper large enough so there is a 1-inch overhang.

Place coconut milk, mango, and sugar in a blender and blend until smooth. Pulse in eggs. Place coconut milk mixture, coconut flour and sesame seeds (if using), in the saucepan with the rice and stir to combine. Pour mixture into prepared baking pan and spread in an even layer. Bake for 40 minutes, or until set. Let cool completely in pan and then lift out using the parchment overhang. Slice into 12 bars and wrap each tightly in foil or other wrapping of choice for transport. Extra cakes can be chilled for up to a week.

GAME CHANGERS Replace canned light coconut milk with carton coconut milk beverage + Swap out coconut sugar for cane sugar

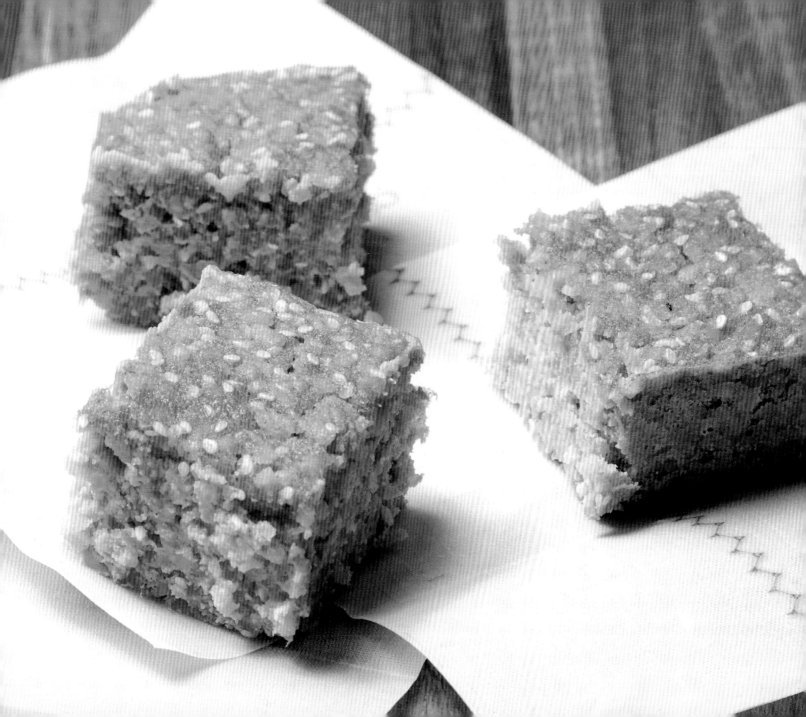

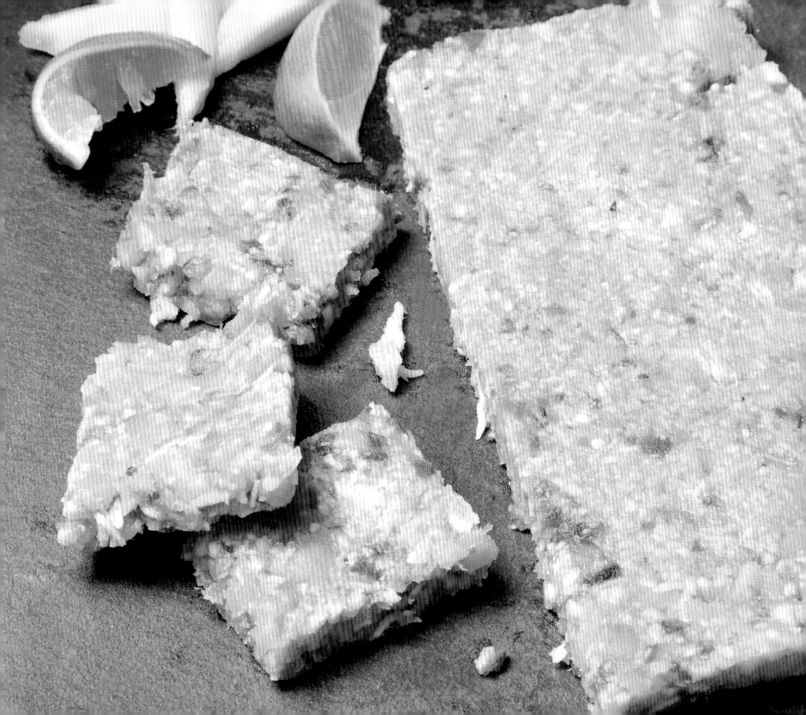

MANGO LIME BARS

A far cry from the dry packaged bars that leave you searching for the nearest spigot, these moist tropical bars deliver plenty of energy from natural sugars to keep you ahead of the pack. Plus, they're fit to eat for all sorts of dietary restrictions.

D F G P V

SERVINGS: 12
ACTIVE TIME: 20 min.

You can also roll the mixture into 1-inch balls for use as a pre-workout nibble or healthy snack.

I keep a few pieces of ginger stashed in the freezer since it's easier to finely grate frozen fresh ginger for use in recipes such as bars and hot drinks.

1½ cups dried mango
1 cup pitted dried dates
1½ cups unsalted dry-roasted cashews
⅓ cup unsweetened shredded coconut
1 teaspoon grated fresh ginger
Zest of 1 lime
⅛ teaspoon salt

Place mango and dates in a bowl, cover with hot water, and let soak for 30 minutes. Drain and pat away excess moisture with paper towels.

Line an 8 × 8–inch square baking pan with a piece of parchment paper large enough so there is a 1-inch overhang. Place cashews in a food processor and process until finely chopped. Add dried fruit, coconut, ginger, lime zest, and salt. Pulse until it sticks together.

Place bar mixture in pan. Place another sheet of parchment paper on top and press down to evenly spread mixture. Leave parchment paper atop and place pan in freezer until bars have hardened, about 2 hours.

Use the parchment paper liner to lift bar mixture out of pan and transfer to a cutting board. Slice into 12 bars and store in an airtight container in the refrigerator for up to 1 week.

GAME CHANGERS Splurge and swap the cashews for macadamia nuts + Replace lime zest with lemon zest

ENDURO BALLS

These are high-calorie, low-volume fuel, which makes them perfect when you are out for the long haul but space is tight—here's looking at you, mountaineers and rock climbers. You can also dole them out as needed during training as a way to customize your calorie intake. A guideline is to pop two balls per hour of activity to help meet your carbohydrate and calorie needs. You can also enjoy the balls prior to a workout to help fuel up for the task ahead.

D F G V

SERVINGS: 18
ACTIVE TIME: 20 min.

The fresh mint seems like an odd addition, but it adds a splash of bright flavor to what can be the standard nut, seed, and dried-fruit energy food combo.

1 cup pitted dates
1½ cups rolled oats
½ cup raw almonds
⅓ cup raw shelled sunflower seeds
¼ cup raw shelled pumpkin seeds (pepitas)
2 tablespoons hemp seeds
2 tablespoons ground flaxseed or ground chia seed (optional)
2 tablespoons cocoa powder
¼ teaspoon salt
⅓ cup honey
¼ cup almond butter
⅓ cup chopped fresh mint
2 teaspoons vanilla extract
⅓ cup mini–chocolate chips (optional)

Soak dates in warm water for 30 minutes. Drain and pat away excess moisture with paper towels.

Place dates, oats, almonds, sunflower seeds, pumpkin seeds, hemp seeds, ground flaxseed or chia (if using), cocoa powder, and salt in a food processor and blend until everything is finely chopped. Add honey, almond butter, mint, and vanilla and blend until the mixture sticks together when pressed between your fingers. Pulse in chocolate chips, if using.

Using slightly damp hands, roll mixture into 1-inch balls. You should have about 18 balls. Store in the refrigerator in an airtight container for up to 1 week.

GAME CHANGERS Use oats labeled "gluten-free" + Replace almonds with pecans + Blend in sesame seeds instead of hemp seeds + Swap out honey for brown rice syrup + Use cashew butter or peanut butter instead of almond butter

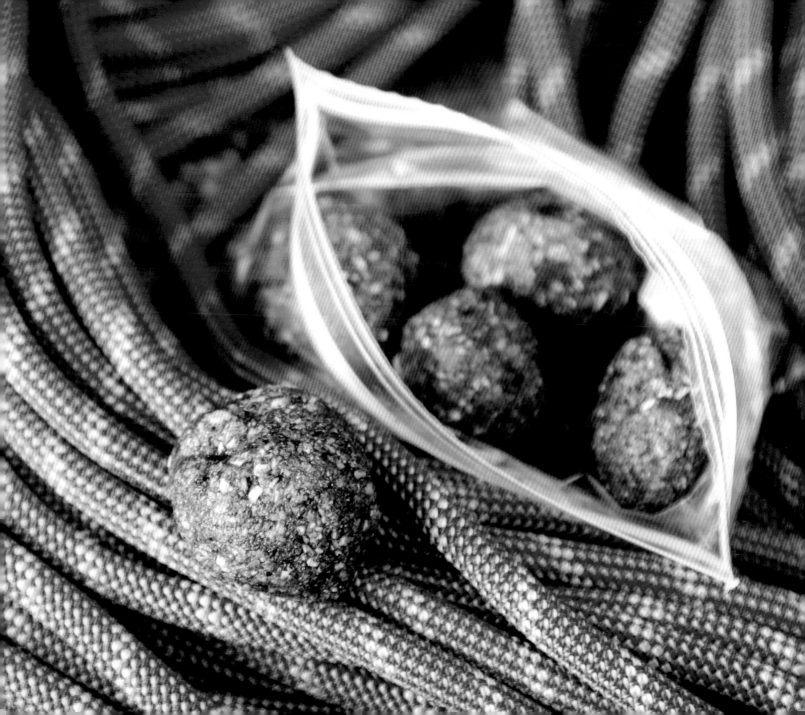

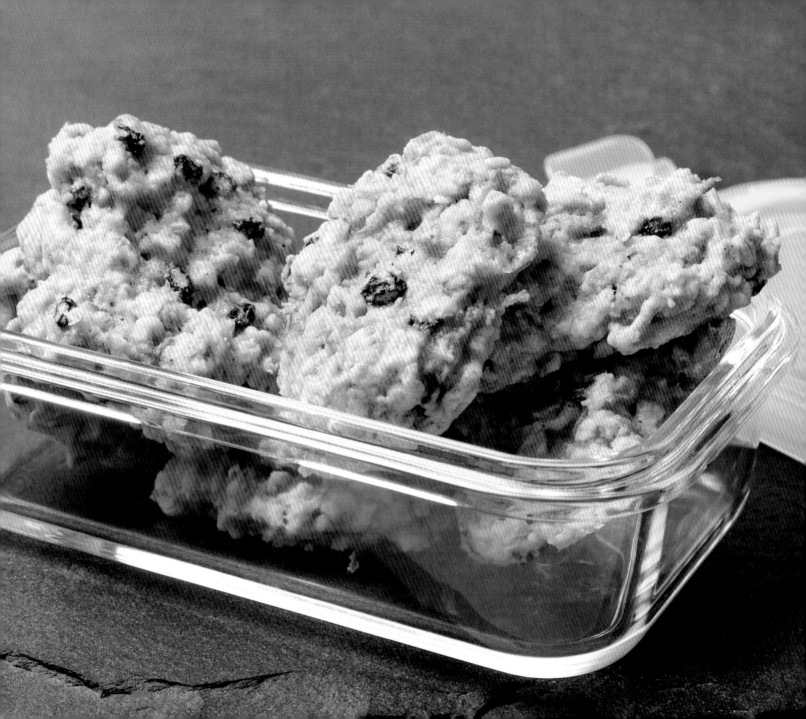

CARROT CAKE COOKIES

It's amazing how something as simple as a homemade cookie can help turn your engine on again when it seems like you're running on fumes. About 75 percent of the calories in each cookie come from carbs, so they can definitely power up your working muscles. Off the bike, I'm not opposed to topping a cookie or two with a slick of cream cheese when a snack craving strikes.

D F G V

SERVINGS: 7
ACTIVE TIME: 20 min.

Chilling the mixture helps the oats soak up some moisture so they don't flatten like a pancake during baking.

To prevent dry and crumbly cookies, level off measurements of oats and flour with the flat side of a knife so you don't add too much.

To quickly raise the temperature of an egg, place it in a bowl of warm water for about 5 minutes.

1 cup quick-cook oats
¾ cup all-purpose flour
1½ teaspoons baking powder
1 teaspoon ground allspice
1 teaspoon ground ginger
¼ teaspoon salt
1 large egg at room temperature
2 tablespoons coconut oil or unsalted butter, melted and cooled slightly
1 teaspoon vanilla extract
½ cup pure maple syrup
¾ cup grated carrot (about 1 medium)
⅓ cup dried currants

In a large bowl, stir together oats, flour, baking powder, allspice, ginger, and salt. In a separate bowl, whisk together egg, oil or butter, and vanilla. Stir in maple syrup. Add wet ingredients to dry ingredients and fold in carrots and currants. Chill mixture for about 30 minutes.

Preheat oven to 325ºF and line a baking sheet with parchment paper or a baking mat. Drop about 14 heaping spoonfuls of batter on the baking sheet, leaving about 1 inch between cookies. Bake for 12 to 15 minutes, or until cookies are still slightly moist to the touch in the center. Cool on baking sheet for a few minutes before cooling completely on wire racks. Chill up to 5 days and transport in small zip-top bags.

GAME CHANGERS Use oats labeled "gluten-free" + Swap out all-purpose flour for oat flour or 1-to-1 gluten-free flour blend + Use cinnamon instead of allspice + Replace maple syrup with honey or agave syrup

FIG CRUMBLE BARS

Fig Newtons have long been a favorite convenience store fuel option for athletes when in need of a blood sugar boost while out on the road. Dense, filling, and chewy, this do-it-yourself version will surely make you the hero of your exercise group. It's perfect energy when you're crushing some calories. If desired, you could work some chopped walnuts into the oat batter.

D G V

SERVINGS: 12
ACTIVE TIME: 25 min.

When adding oils to bar recipes such as these, you'll want to use one with a neutral flavor (canola, sunflower, light olive, or grapeseed) so it doesn't impact the taste of the final product.

2 cups dried Mission figs, stems trimmed
1 cup apple juice
1 tablespoon lemon zest
2 cups all-purpose flour
1 cup rolled oats
2 tablespoons ground flaxseed
1½ teaspoons cinnamon
1 teaspoon baking soda
¼ teaspoon salt
½ cup canola, sunflower, light olive, or grapeseed oil
½ cup unsweetened applesauce
⅓ cup honey

Place figs, apple juice, lemon zest, and a pinch of salt in a medium-sized saucepan. Bring to a boil, reduce heat to low, and simmer, covered, for 20 minutes. Remove from heat, uncover, and let cool for about 15 minutes. Place figs and any remaining liquid in a food processor and puree.

Preheat oven to 350°F. Line an 8 × 8–inch square baking pan with a piece of parchment paper large enough so there is a 1-inch overhang. In a large bowl, stir together flour, oats, flaxseed, cinnamon, baking soda, and salt. In a separate bowl, stir together oil, applesauce, and honey. Add wet ingredients to dry ingredients and mix until everything is moist.

Place half of the oat mixture in the prepared pan and press down firmly to form a compact, even layer. Scoop fig puree on top and spread out into an even layer. Place the remainder of the oat mixture over the figs and spread out into an even layer. Bake for 25 minutes, or until the edges are golden. Let cool completely in the pan before lifting out using the parchment overhang and slicing into 12 bars. Chill for up to 1 week and wrap tightly in foil or other wrapping of choice for transport.

GAME CHANGERS Swap out lemon zest for orange zest + Try oat flour or spelt flour in lieu of all-purpose flour + Use oats labeled "gluten-free" and replace the all-purpose flour with a 1-to-1 gluten-free flour blend + Use ground chia seed instead of flaxseed + Replace the oil with melted coconut oil + Sweeten with brown rice syrup or agave syrup instead of honey

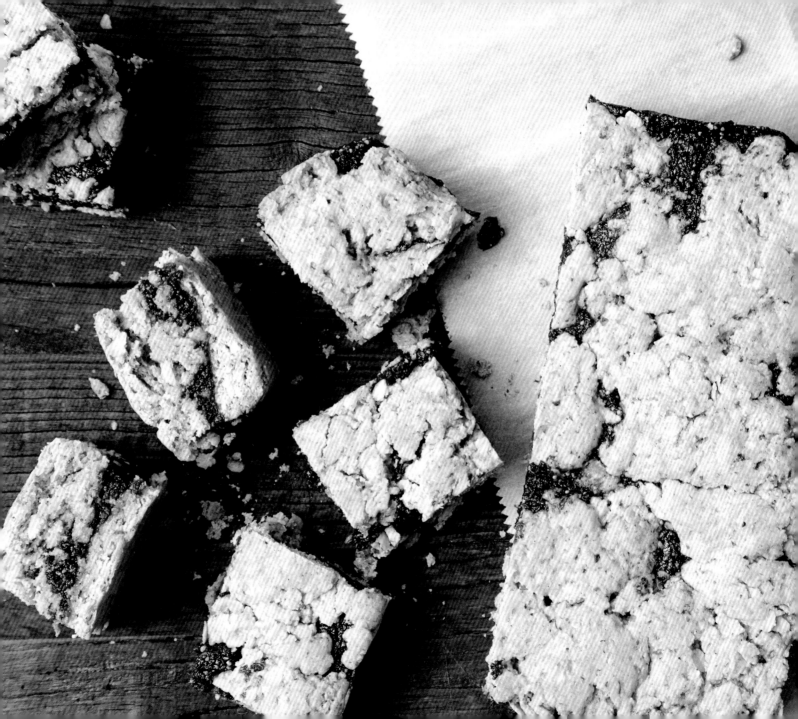

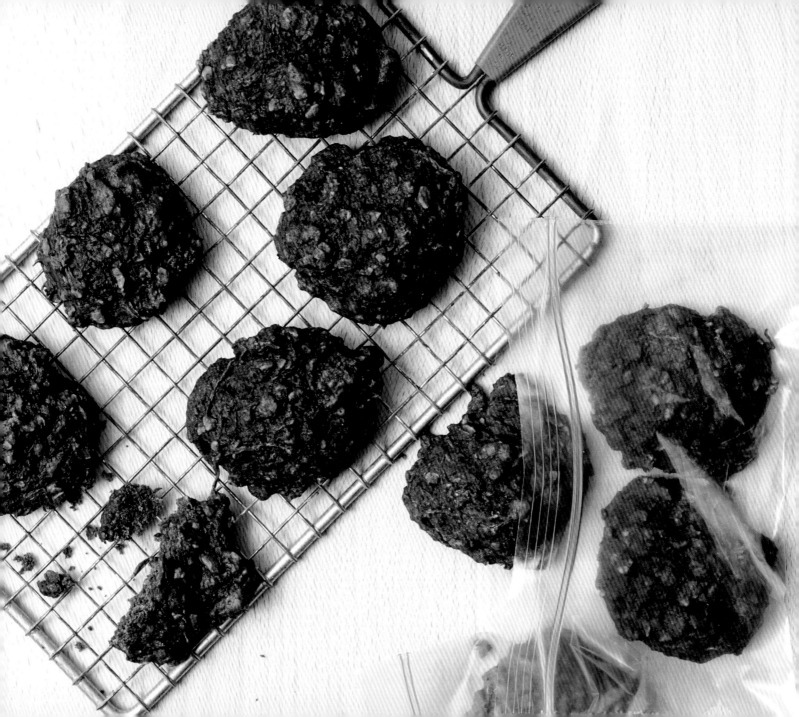

ZUCCHINI BREAD BITES

Here's how to transform tender zucchini bread into a transportable source of appetizing carbohydrate fuel. You can also stir some chopped walnuts into the batter or, for a little kick, try mixing in about ¼ teaspoon of chili powder.

D F G V

SERVINGS: 12
ACTIVE TIME: 25 min.

For ease of digestion, I often use refined all-purpose flour for recipes such as this that are meant to be consumed during activity. However, my other baking almost always focuses on more nutrient-dense whole-grain flours such as whole wheat pastry flour. Feel free to experiment with other flours to see what works best for you.

1 cup finely grated zucchini
1 cup all-purpose flour
¾ cup quinoa flakes
3 tablespoons cocoa powder
1 teaspoon cinnamon
1 teaspoon ground ginger (optional)
½ teaspoon salt
¾ teaspoon baking powder
½ teaspoon baking soda
1 large egg
½ cup unsweetened applesauce
⅓ cup pure maple syrup
3 tablespoons melted and cooled coconut oil
1 teaspoon vanilla extract

Place zucchini in a colander, sprinkle on a couple pinches of salt, and let sit 15 minutes. Using your hands, squeeze out as much moisture as possible.

Preheat oven to 375ºF. In a large bowl, stir together flour, quinoa flakes, cocoa powder, cinnamon, ground ginger (if using), salt, baking powder, and baking soda. In a separate bowl, whisk together egg, applesauce, maple syrup, coconut oil, and vanilla. Add wet ingredients to dry ingredients and mix gently. Fold in zucchini.

Line a baking sheet with parchment paper or a silicone baking mat. By the tablespoonful, place batter on the baking sheet. You should get about 24 balls. Bake until edges are browned and tops give slightly when pressed gently, about 12 minutes. Allow to cool completely, preferably on metal racks. Chill for up to 5 days and transport in a small zip-top bag.

GAME CHANGERS Replace all-purpose flour with oat flour, spelt flour, or 1-to-1 gluten-free flour blend ✦ Try quick-cook oats or millet flakes instead of quinoa flakes ✦ Use a neutral-tasting oil like canola or grapeseed instead of coconut

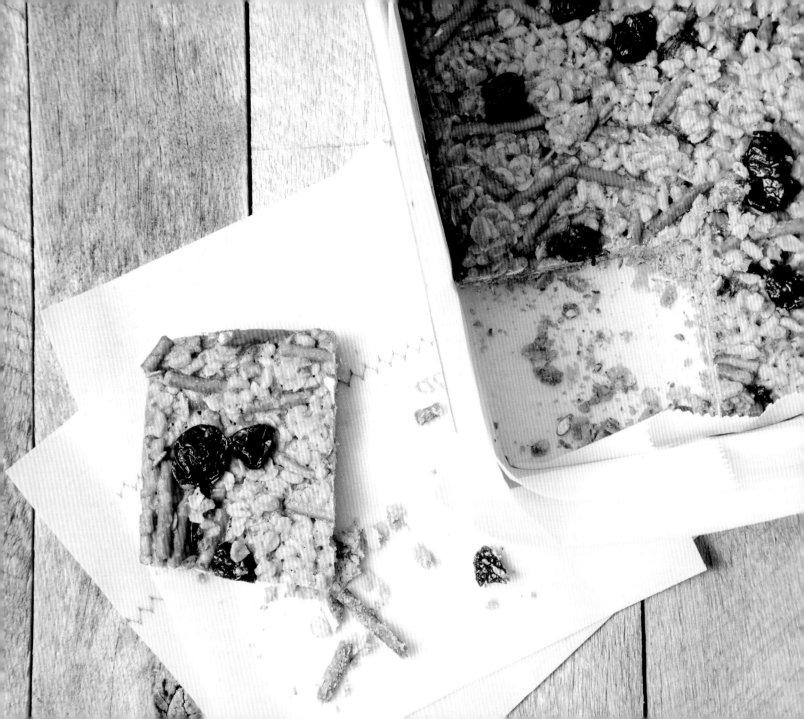

PEANUT PRETZEL SQUARES

If I was to make my own cycling jersey, it could very well say "Will pedal for Peanut Pretzel Squares." These squares have a winning mix of salty crunch, energizing carbs, and peanut butter goodness to keep your palate and muscles feeling rewarded.

D F G V

SERVINGS: 12
ACTIVE TIME: 20 min.

Good peanut butter should just be, well, peanuts! So look for a brand that does not include any added sugar or dreaded hydrogenated oil. Often, these nut butters are labeled "natural."

1½ cups roughly chopped salted pretzel sticks
1 cup rolled oats
1 cup puffed rice cereal
¼ cup all-purpose flour
3 tablespoons ground flaxseed
⅔ cup smooth peanut butter
½ cup honey
3 tablespoons coconut oil
½ cup dried cherries (optional)

Preheat oven to 325°F. Line an 8 × 8–inch square baking pan with a piece of parchment paper large enough so there is a 1-inch overhang.

In a large bowl, stir together pretzels, oats, puffed rice, flour, and flaxseed.

Place peanut butter, honey, and coconut oil in a small saucepan. Heat over medium until the mixture is fluid, about 3 minutes. Mix peanut butter mixture into oat mixture until everything is moist. Stir in cherries, if using.

Place mixture in pan and spread out in an even layer.

Bake for 20 minutes, or until edges are golden. Let cool in pan completely, carefully lift out of pan using parchment overhang and slice into 12 squares. If you find the bars are crumbling during cutting, stick the mixture in the fridge to chill for several minutes and then try again. Keep chilled for up to 5 days or freeze extras for up to 1 month.

GAME CHANGERS Use gluten-free pretzels, oats labeled "gluten-free," and 1-to-1 gluten-free flour blend instead of all-purpose flour + Replace oats with quinoa, spelt, or barley flakes + Swap out ground flaxseed for ground chia seed + Try almond butter in lieu of peanut butter + Use brown rice syrup instead of honey + Replace coconut oil with unsalted butter

GRANOLA BITES

Who says granola has to be served in a bowl? These little bundles of nutrients are an on-the-go way to carry your beloved hippie food. You will be perfectly happy getting lost in the woods or stuck on the steepest of inclines if you have these nearby.

D F G V

SERVINGS: 12
ACTIVE TIME: 20 min.

You can also make these in regular-sized muffin cups for a more substantial post-workout nosh or a take-and-go breakfast option. Just increase cooking time by about 5 minutes.

1½ cups quick-cook oats
⅓ cup wheat germ
½ cup chopped pecans or almonds
¼ cup hemp seeds
½ cup dried cranberries
½ cup chopped dried apricots
⅓ cup unsweetened shredded coconut
½ teaspoon cinnamon
½ teaspoon ground ginger
½ teaspoon salt
1 large egg
½ cup honey or brown rice syrup
¼ cup melted coconut oil

Preheat oven to 350°F. In a large bowl, stir together oats, wheat germ, pecans or almonds, hemp seeds, cranberries, apricots, coconut, cinnamon, ginger, and salt. In a separate bowl, lightly beat egg and stir in honey or brown rice syrup and oil. Add wet ingredients to dry and mix until everything is moist.

Divide mixture among 24 greased or paper-lined mini-muffin cups and make sure to pack it down tightly to help hold everything together. Bake for 15 minutes, or until the edges begin to brown. Let cool several minutes before unmolding. Chill in the refrigerator for up to 1 week and transport in a small zip-top bag.

GAME CHANGERS Use oats labeled "gluten-free" or replace oats with quinoa flakes, barley flakes, or spelt flakes + Use almond flour or ground flaxseed instead of wheat germ + Stir in sunflower seeds instead of hemp seeds + Swap out cranberries for dried cherries, chopped dried pineapple, or goji berries

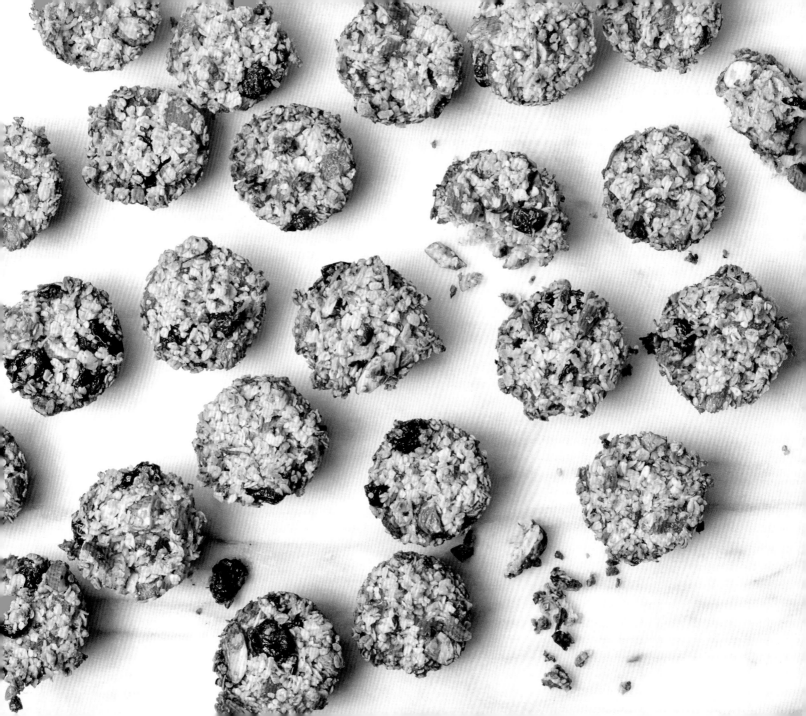

MEDITERRANEAN MINI MUFFINS

Inhale one of these bite-sized muffins, close your eyes, and imagine you're cycling in the Italian countryside, running on a white sand Mediterranean beach, or hiking in the towering French Alps. OK, so your workout or race might be more pedestrian, but these mini-muffins offer a welcome respite from sweet, sugary calories. They also deliver a shot of salt for those times when you need to replace some lost sodium.

D F G V

SERVINGS: 12
ACTIVE TIME: 20 min.

You can also make these in standard-sized muffin cups for an anytime snack or even as a dinner side dish served warm with a slick of butter. You'll need to increase the cooking time by about 5 minutes. You can also up the nutritional ante by using whole-grain flour such as whole wheat pastry flour or spelt flour if ease of digestion during exercise is not a concern.

1¾ cups all-purpose flour
¼ cup finely ground cornmeal
3 tablespoons sugar
1½ teaspoons baking powder
1 teaspoon dried thyme
½ teaspoon salt
2 large eggs
¾ cup + 2 tablespoons low-fat milk
⅓ cup olive oil
   Zest of 1 lemon (optional)
2 ounces finely chopped feta cheese (about ½ cup)
½ cup drained and finely chopped roasted red bell peppers
⅓ cup pitted, finely chopped Kalamata olives

Preheat oven to 350ºF. In a large bowl, mix together flour, cornmeal, sugar, baking powder, thyme, and salt. In a separate bowl, whisk together eggs, milk, oil, and lemon zest, if using. Add wet ingredients to dry ingredients and mix gently until flour is incorporated Fold in feta, red peppers, and olives.

Divide among 24 greased or paper-lined mini-muffin cups and bake for 15 minutes, or until a toothpick inserted into the center of a muffin comes out mostly clean. Let cool for a few minutes before unmolding and cooling completely on metal racks. Keep chilled for up to 5 days and transport in small zip-top bags.

GAME CHANGERS Use 1-to-1 gluten-free flour blend instead of all-purpose flour ✦ Make these dairy-free with nondairy milk and no feta ✦ Try grapeseed oil or canola oil instead of olive oil ✦ Use chopped sun-dried tomatoes instead of roasted peppers

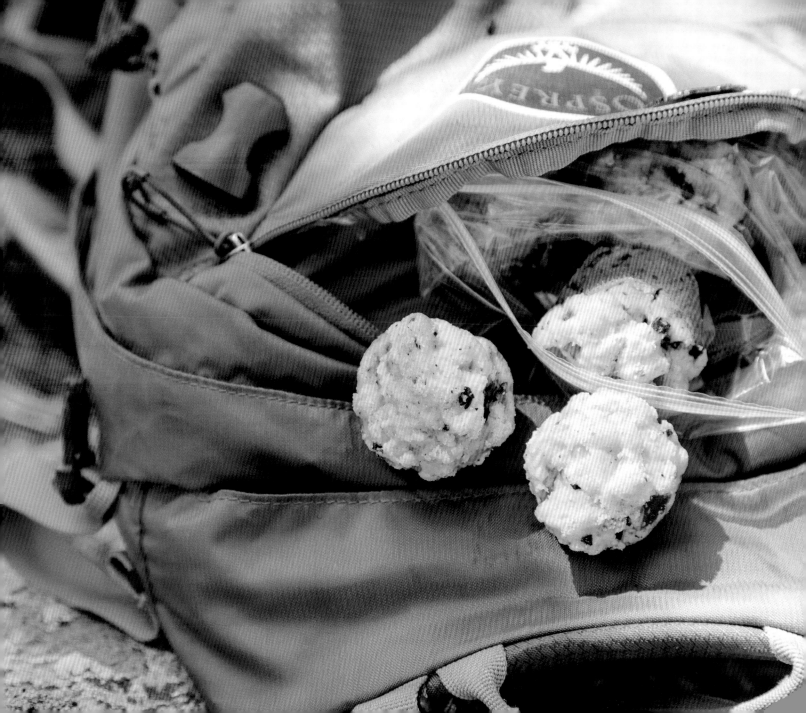

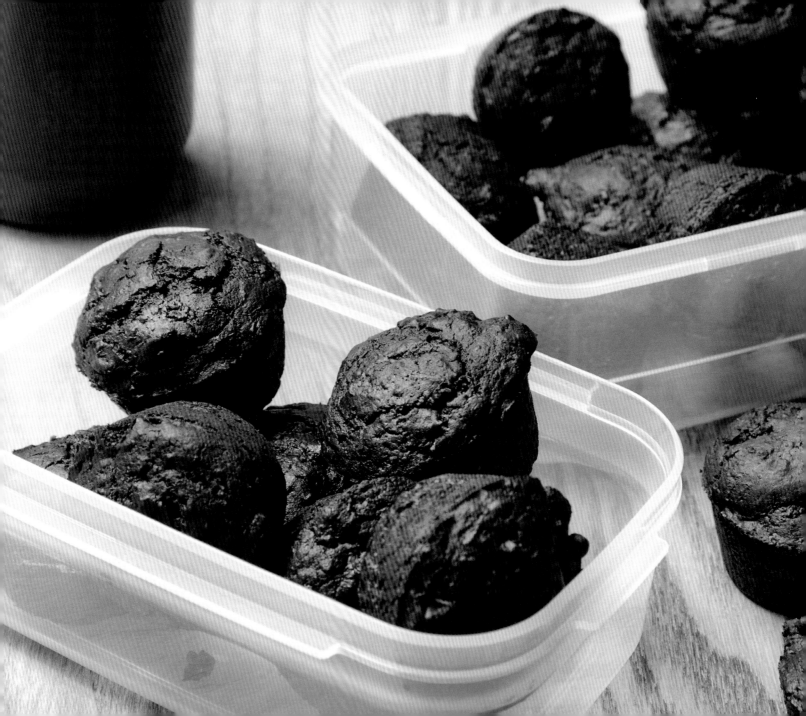

BROWNIE BITES

Butternut squash is the stealth ingredient in these two-bite brownies. It provides natural sweetness and also lets you cut back on the amount of fat needed, making these treats easier to digest when you're about to push the pace. I especially like taking these along on sultry days, when they become even more fudgelike as they warm in my jersey pocket. They're also great to take to potlucks.

D F G V

SERVINGS: 10
ACTIVE TIME: 20 min.

If you're looking for a shortcut, head to the baby food section and look for jars or squeeze pouches of pureed butternut squash or sweet potato (no other ingredients). Use the equivalent of 8 ounces of puree in this recipe. Some grocers also carry pre-cut, peeled butternut squash.

If using darker Dutch-processed cocoa instead of unsweetened (natural), replace the baking soda with baking powder.

½ pound peeled and diced butternut squash (about 2 cups)
¼ cup melted unsalted butter or melted coconut oil
2 large eggs, lightly beaten
⅔ cup unsweetened cocoa powder
½ cup coconut sugar, turbinado sugar, or brown sugar
2 teaspoons vanilla extract
½ cup all-purpose flour
1 teaspoon cinnamon
½ teaspoon baking soda
¼ teaspoon salt

Preheat oven to 350°F.

Steam or boil squash until fork-tender. Place cooked squash in a bowl and mash until smooth. Add the butter or coconut oil, eggs, cocoa powder, sugar, and vanilla to the squash mixture and mix. In a separate bowl, mix together the flour, cinnamon, baking soda, and salt. Stir the squash mixture into the flour mixture and mix just until no dry parts are visible.

Divide mixture among 20 silicone or greased or paper-lined metal mini-muffin cups. Bake for 15 minutes, or until a toothpick inserted into the center of a brownie comes out nearly clean. Let cool for a few minutes before unmolding and cooling completely on metal racks. Chill for up to 5 days and transport in small zip-top bags.

GAME CHANGERS Use pureed sweet potato instead of squash + Make these whole grain by using oat flour, spelt flour, or whole wheat pastry flour + Use 1-to-1 gluten-free flour blend instead of all-purpose flour + Add a fiery kick by blending in ¼ teaspoon chili powder

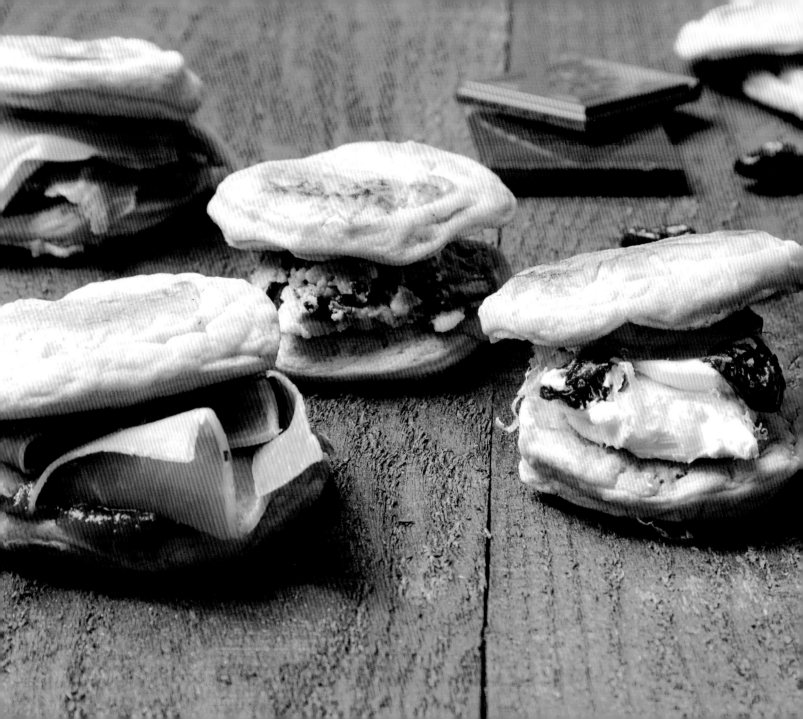

BLINI SLIDERS

Blini are essentially tiny pancakes hailing from Russia that are often served as a fanciful appetizer adorned with caviar. But they can be stuffed with all sorts of tasty combos for whimsical mini-sandwiches that are neat little packages of fuel. Of course, you can also go old school and simply slather on PB&J. I also switch things up by using other flours such as oat, spelt, brown rice, or even almond.

SERVINGS: 12
ACTIVE TIME: 20 min.

This batter can be used to make a stack of larger-sized breakfast pancakes.

The batter can be mixed together up to 24 hours in advance if covered and chilled. The blinis themselves can be made up to 5 days in advance (and frozen for future use if tightly wrapped), but Sliders are best assembled the day of consumption.

BLINI
- 1 cup all-purpose flour or 1-to-1 gluten-free flour blend
- ½ teaspoon baking powder
- ½ teaspoon baking soda
- 2 large eggs
- ¾ cup milk or unflavored nondairy milk
- 1 tablespoon butter or oil such as canola or coconut

COCO CHOCO
- ⅓ cup coconut butter (not coconut oil)
- 2 ounces chopped dark chocolate

APPLE PORK
- ⅓ cup apple butter
- 3 ounces prosciutto, roughly chopped

CHERRY CHEESECAKE
- ⅓ cup reduced-fat cream cheese
- ½ cup dried cherries
- Zest of 1 lemon

Combine flour, baking powder, baking soda, and a pinch of salt in a large bowl. In a separate bowl, gently beat together eggs and milk. Add wet ingredients to dry ingredients and stir until smooth. Let batter rest 10 minutes. The mixture should be the consistency of pancake batter, so add additional milk, 1 tablespoon at a time, if it's too thick.

Heat butter or oil in a skillet over medium heat. By the tablespoonful, drop batter into pan and heat mini-pancakes until edges begin to brown and bubbles form on the surface, about 2 to 3 minutes. Flip over and cook for 2 minutes more, or until golden brown on the bottom. Repeat with remaining batter, adding more butter or oil to pan as needed. Let prepared blini cool, preferably on a wire rack. You should get at least 22 mini-pancakes.

To assemble, divide one of the flavor combinations below among half of the blini and then top with remaining blini to form mini-pancake sandwiches. To transport, wrap tightly in a piece of foil or other wrapping of choice.

HAND PIES

Cycling down the iconic Ruta 40 in Argentina became a whole lot tastier when my girlfriend and I discovered that the handheld pies known as empanadas make for stellar on-the-go fuel. After extensive sampling, we deemed Caprese our favorite flavor, but the great thing with empanadas, as these incarnations demonstrate, is that they are so versatile. They can be stuffed with all sorts of sweet and savory combinations, making every outing a new gastronomic delight.

SERVINGS: 8
ACTIVE TIME: 25 min.

Frozen pie shells are a convenient way to get the job done fast, but no amount of exercise can cancel out eating trans fat, so make sure the ingredient list is free of hydrogenated oil or shortening. You can also scour Google for DIY empanada crusts or look for pre-made empanada rounds at Latin grocers.

2 frozen pie shells, defrosted at room temperature
1 egg

NUTTY MANGO
¼ cup cashew butter
¼ cup mango chutney

CAPRESE
1 cup grated mozzarella cheese
1 cup quartered cherry tomatoes
⅓ cup chopped fresh basil

SAVORY APPLE PIE
1 apple, finely chopped
4 ounces grated cheddar cheese (about 1 cup)
1 tablespoon finely chopped rosemary

Preheat oven to 375°F. Working with one pie shell at a time, flip shell and its container upside down on a lightly floured work surface, carefully release pie shell from container, and press down gently to flatten. If any cracks form, seal shut with moistened fingers. Slice pie shell into 4 equal-sized triangles. Whisk egg with 1 tablespoon water.

Place some of one of the filling combinations in the center of each triangle. Do not overstuff. Brush edges with the egg wash, fold one end of each triangle over to form a smaller triangle, and seal each shut with the tines of a fork. Place pies on a baking sheet lined with parchment paper or a silicone baking mat and brush tops with more egg wash. Repeat with remaining pie shell and filling.

Bake for 15 minutes, or until golden brown. Let cool completely before storing in the refrigerator for up to 5 days. Transport pies in small zip-top bags.

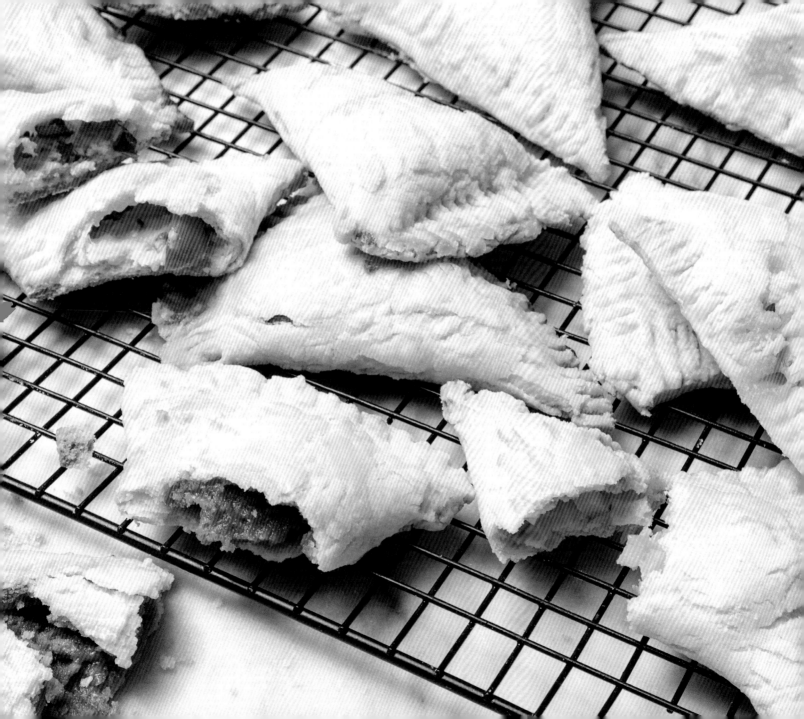

CREPE ROLLS

Not just for Sunday brunch, crepes are a great way to roll up all sorts of filling combinations in a highly transportable package. And making crepes is not nearly the high-flying kitchen feat it's made out to be. The flavors below will guarantee one of your tastiest exercise sessions ever, but there is also nothing wrong with a comforting combination of peanut butter and jam. You can bring a few different crepe combinations on long outings to keep your palate guessing.

D F G V

SERVINGS: 8
ACTIVE TIME: 35 min.

The batter can be mixed together up to 24 hours in advance if covered and chilled. The crepes themselves can be made up to 4 days in advance, but are best stuffed and rolled the day of consumption.

CREPES

1 cup all-purpose flour or 1-to-1 gluten-free flour blend

2 large eggs, lightly beaten

1 cup low-fat milk or plain nondairy milk

¼ cup water

¼ teaspoon salt

2 tablespoons neutral-tasting oil, such as grapeseed, canola, or light olive

PAD THAI

SPREAD*

6 tablespoons peanut butter

2 tablespoons soy sauce

1 teaspoon sriracha

1 teaspoon ground ginger

Juice of ½ lime

* Stir ingredients together in small bowl

TOPPING

3 ounces cold cooked soba noodles or wide rice noodles

1 large carrot, shredded

½ cup cilantro

HAWAIIAN PIZZA

SPREAD

½ cup tomato sauce

TOPPING

8 thin slices ham, about 8 ounces

1½ cups diced pineapple

1 cup shredded mozzarella

CHOCOLATY BANANA

SPREAD

⅓ cup almond butter

TOPPING

2 medium-sized bananas, thinly sliced

¼ cup chocolate chips

Place batter ingredients in a blender and blend until smooth. Alternatively, whisk together the ingredients in a large bowl until no lumps are present. The batter should be thin.

Heat an 8- to 10-inch cast-iron or nonstick skillet over medium heat until a drop of water sizzles on the surface. Be sure to grease pan with oil or butter if not completely nonstick. Pour ¼ cup batter into pan

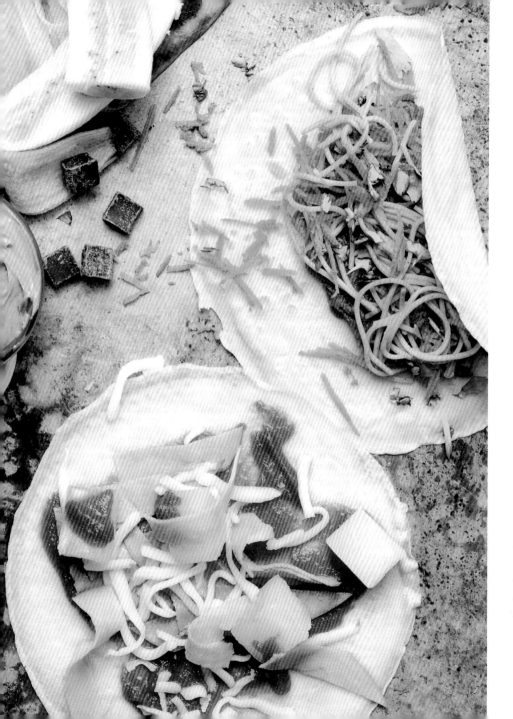

and quickly lift the skillet off the burner, then tilt and swirl the pan so the batter forms a large thin circle. Place pan back on heat and cook for 2 minutes, or until edges begin to turn golden brown, the center has dried, and the crepe blisters on the bottom. Loosen with a thin spatula, flip, and cook the other side for 30 seconds.

Slide the crepe out of the skillet and repeat with remaining batter to make at least 8 crepes. To minimize risk of tearing, let crepes cool for an hour, ideally on metal racks, before filling. Do not stack crepes while they are cooling or they may become soggy. For later use, wrap stacked crepes in foil or plastic wrap and store in the refrigerator.

To assemble, slather one of the spreads over most of the crepe. Apply topping to bottom third of crepes, and tightly roll, tucking in ingredients as needed. Keep whole or slice in half. To transport, tightly wrap in aluminum foil or other wrap of choice. To freeze for future use, separate each crepe with parchment or waxed paper and place in an airtight container. Crepes can be frozen for up to 3 months, but let them thaw completely before separating.

PLANTAIN RICE WRAPS

Plantains, the giant of the banana world, are deliciously sweet when ripe, and when paired with rice and a tortilla will flood your bloodstream with energy-boosting carbs. If desired, top the plantain mash with a dusting of cinnamon, a drizzle of molasses or honey, or a scatting of raisins before rolling. You can even turn these into a lunch or post-workout repast by topping with some canned black beans and salsa.

D F G V

SERVINGS: 6
ACTIVE TIME: 15 min.

Use plantains that have a significant amount of black on their skin, which indicates that they are at their sweetest. To peel a plantain, slice off about ½ inch from each end, run a sharp knife down the length of the fruit, and then peel back the skin.

Extra rice and plantain mixture can be frozen separately for future wraps.

2 ripe plantains, sliced
Juice of 1 lime
Zest of 1 lime
½ teaspoon ground ginger (optional)
¾ cup white jasmine rice
1½ cups coconut water
6 8-inch tortillas

Place plantains, lime juice, and ½ cup water in a small saucepan. Bring to a boil, reduce heat to medium-low, and simmer until plantains are very tender. Stir in lime zest, ginger (if using), and a pinch of salt and then mash with a fork or potato masher.

Place rice and coconut water in a separate saucepan. Bring to a boil, reduce heat to medium-low, and simmer, covered, until rice is tender and coconut water has been absorbed, about 15 minutes. Remove from heat, let rest, covered, for 5 minutes, and then fluff with a fork.

For each wrap, place some rice on a tortilla and top with some mashed plantain. Don't overstuff. Tightly roll and wrap in foil or place in small zip-top bag for transport.

GAME CHANGERS Replace jasmine rice with basmati rice + Use gluten-free wraps

STRAWBERRY CHEESECAKE WRAPS

Here's a way to combine your love of adventure with satisfying a craving for dessert. Each serving delivers plenty of carbs to help blast you to the finish line or postcard-worthy viewpoint. For a pre-workout or post-workout snack, replace the tortilla with rice cakes.

SERVINGS: 6
ACTIVE TIME: 15 min.

Made by whipping it into a more spreadable product, whipped cream cheese is an easier option to work with than regular cream cheese for items such as wraps and rice cakes.

2 cups fresh or frozen (thawed) strawberries
3 Medjool dates, pitted
1 tablespoon fresh lemon juice
4 teaspoons chia seeds
1 cup whipped cream cheese
2 teaspoons lemon zest
1 teaspoon vanilla extract
6 8-inch tortillas
⅓ cup chopped fresh mint (optional)

Using a blender or food processor, puree together strawberries, dates, and lemon juice. Place mixture in a container and stir in chia seeds. Cover and chill to thicken for at least 1 hour or up to 3 days.

Stir together whipped cream cheese, lemon zest, and vanilla. Keep chilled until ready to use, for up to 5 days.

To assemble, spread some cream cheese mixture on a tortilla and top with strawberry puree and mint, if using. Tightly roll wrap in foil or place in small zip-top bags for transport.

GAME CHANGERS Swap out strawberries for raspberries + Replace lemon juice and zest with lime + Use gluten-free wraps + Use fresh basil instead of mint

SUSHI ROLLS

If you're looking for portable fuel that offers a change of pace, don't overlook the egg roll wrapper. Easy to fill and roll, when baked they hold together very well, even on bumpy terrain. And the filling options are almost endless, so once you get comfortable with this sushi-inspired one, feel free to play around with all sorts of savory and sweet combos.

SERVINGS: 5
ACTIVE TIME: 25 min.

Not to be confused with smaller wonton wrappers, egg roll wrappers can be found in most supermarkets, often near the produce aisle.

1 cup cooked short-grain or medium-grain white rice
1 (5-ounce) can tuna, drained and broken into chunks
2 chopped nori sheets
⅓ cup chopped pickled ginger
3 tablespoons reduced-sodium soy sauce
1½ tablespoons rice vinegar
10 egg roll wrappers

Preheat oven to 375°F. In a bowl, stir together white rice, tuna, nori, pickled ginger, soy sauce, and rice vinegar.

Place an egg roll wrapper on a flat work surface with a corner pointing toward you. Scoop about 2 tablespoons of the tuna mixture onto the center of the wrap. Brush the top and bottom corners of the wrap with water, and fold the bottom corner of the egg roll wrapper over the tuna stuffing to meet the top corner, creating a triangle. Brush the two outside corners with water and fold

them in toward the center. Roll tightly from the long bottom edge up toward the remaining triangle point at the top. Place seam-side down on a baking sheet lined with parchment paper or a silicone baking mat. Repeat with remaining tuna mixture and egg roll wraps. Brush tops with oil. Bake for 15 minutes, flip, and bake for an additional 5 minutes. Let cool to room temperature, preferably on a metal rack, before storing in the refrigerator for up to 5 days. Transport in small zip-top bags.

GAME CHANGERS Try black rice instead of white rice
✦ Replace tuna with canned salmon ✦ Use tamari or liquid aminos instead of soy sauce

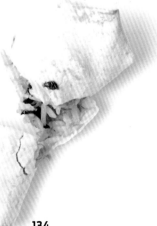

MAPLE APPLESAUCE ROLLS

These highly portable rolls are plush with energizing carbs and are akin to apple turnovers. What's great is that you won't need to roll out pie dough or make a pit stop at a bakery. Heck, you could make a case for serving these warm with a scoop or two of ice cream as a dessert.

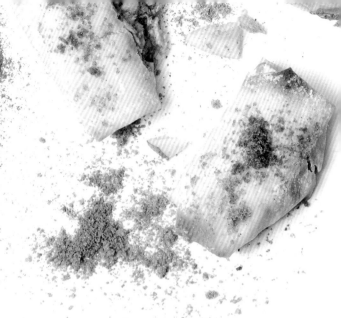

SERVINGS: 5
ACTIVE TIME: 25 min.

If you can't find graham cracker crumbs, simply take whole graham crackers and crush them in a food processor, with a mortar and pestle, or in a zip-top bag using a rolling pin.

3 apples, peeled, cored, and roughly chopped
¼ cup graham cracker crumbs
3 tablespoons pure maple syrup
   Juice of ½ lemon
¾ teaspoon cinnamon, divided
¼ teaspoon nutmeg
1 tablespoon brown sugar or coconut sugar
10 egg roll wrappers
1 tablespoon melted butter

Preheat oven to 375°F. Place apples, graham cracker crumbs, maple syrup, lemon juice, ½ teaspoon cinnamon, nutmeg, and a pinch of salt in a food processor and blend until the mixture is slightly chunky. Stir together sugar and ¼ teaspoon cinnamon; set aside.

Place an egg roll wrapper on a flat work surface and scoop about 2 tablespoons of the apple mixture onto the center of the wrap. Fold two corners of the egg roll wrapper over the apple stuffing so that the tips touch each other. Brush the other corners with water and fold in toward the center. Roll tightly from the bottom up. Place seam-side down on a baking sheet lined with parchment paper or a silicone baking mat. Repeat with remaining apple mixture and egg roll wrappers. Brush tops with half of the butter. Bake for 15 minutes and then brush with remaining butter and sprinkle cinnamon sugar over tops. Bake for an additional 5 minutes, or until crispy. Let cool to room temperature, preferably on a metal rack, before storing in the refrigerator for up to 5 days. Transport in small zip-top bags.

GAME CHANGERS Swap out apple for a slightly underripe pear + Use almond flour or hazelnut flour instead of graham cracker crumbs + Replace cinnamon and nutmeg with pumpkin pie spice

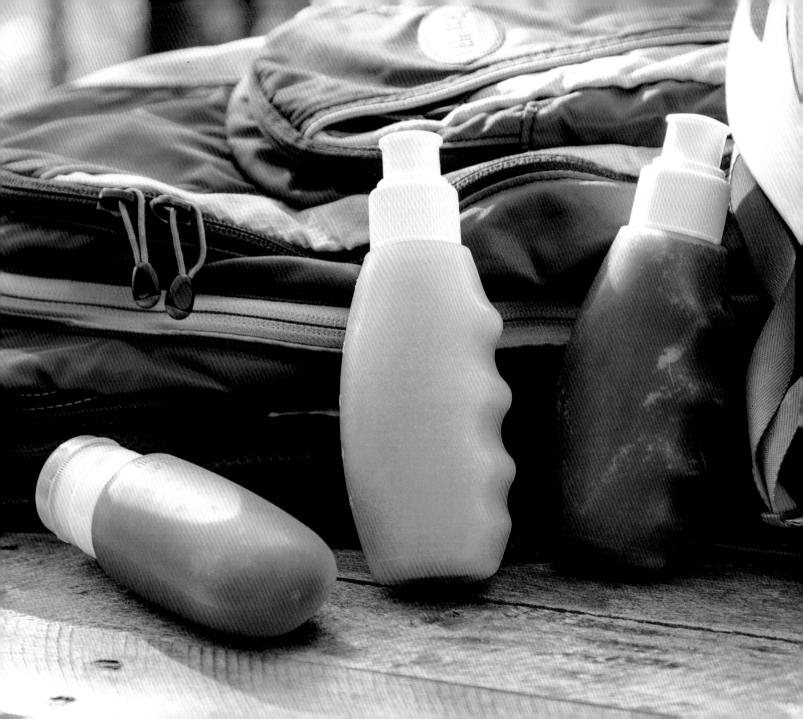

ENERGY SHOTS

When you're going hard for a long time, you're going to hit a wall at some point. Rather than waiting for your blood sugar to take a nosedive, try one of these economical, fruity energy shots instead of a messy packaged gel. The au naturel sugars in dried fruit will give you that much-needed quick blast of energy, particularly if you are struggling to chew and swallow solids as the pace increases. The combination of glucose and fructose in dried fruit also increases carb absorption rates during exercise and can lead to fewer gastrointestinal issues. Keep in mind, however, that taking in highly concentrated carbohydrates during activity can force water from your blood into your digestive tract to help dilute the solution to better match body fluid osmolality, an outcome that may lead to stomach woes and heightened risk for dehydration. So these energy shots are best chased with some water (about 4 ounces) to help encourage absorption and hydration.

SERVINGS: 2
ACTIVE TIME: 5 min.

For a cheap alternative to dedicated gel flasks, consider looking in the personal care section of retailers, where you'll likely find little travel accessory bottles. They can serve the same function at a more budget-friendly price.

For a caffeinated flavor choice, see the Energy Jolt option on page 71.

BERRY MAPLE

⅓ cup dried blueberries
⅔ cup boiling water
2 tablespoons pure maple syrup
½ teaspoon lemon zest
⅛ teaspoon salt

HONEY OF AN APRICOT

⅓ cup dried apricots
¾ cup boiling water
1 tablespoon honey
⅛ teaspoon ground ginger
⅛ teaspoon salt

PERKY RAISIN

⅓ cup raisins
¾ cup boiling water
2 tablespoons brown sugar or coconut sugar
1 teaspoon unsweetened cocoa powder

1 teaspoon instant espresso powder
½ teaspoon vanilla extract
⅛ teaspoon salt

PB&J

⅓ cup dried cherries
¾ cup boiling water
1 tablespoon smooth peanut butter
2 teaspoons honey
⅛ teaspoon salt (omit if using salted peanut butter)

Place dried fruit and boiling water in a blender container and let soak for 30 minutes. Add remaining ingredients and blend until as smooth as possible. Let cool and then transfer to one large gel flask or two smaller ones. These can be made a day in advance and kept chilled until use.

SPORTS DRINKS

A well-designed sports drink can provide an important mix of fluid, fast-digesting carbs, and electrolytes to help keep you going. These combos make enough to fill a 24-ounce (3-cup) water bottle, so double or triple the recipe if you want to fill multiple bottles. They're designed to have no more than 5 percent carbohydrate concentration (5 grams per 100 mL) to help maximize stomach emptying and intestinal absorption by being hypotonic—at a slightly lower carb content than your body fluid to encourage your cells to absorb the liquid faster than they do plain water or drinks with a higher carb percentage. The combination of glucose and fructose in these drinks also helps promote absorption for better performance and less chance of an unhappy gut. The recipes supply about 145 mg of sodium per cup, more than most commercial sports drinks but still on the lower end of concentration in lost sweat. This is to take into account extra sodium you may obtain from other fuel sources during exercise. But assess your situation—you can always add a pinch or two of extra salt.

SERVINGS: 1
ACTIVE TIME: 5 min.

Studies have found that sipping cold fluids during endurance exercise can improve performance, likely by helping lower your core temperature. So when temps are soaring, make an extra half-batch of a sports drink and freeze it as ice cubes. Then pop a few of the ice cubes into your bottle with the sports drink.

CIDERADE

1¾ cups water

1¼ cups pure apple cider

¼ teaspoon cinnamon

⅛ teaspoon + ¹⁄₁₆ teaspoon sea salt

MAPLE ORANGE

2 cups water

1 cup pulp-free orange juice

2 tablespoons pure maple syrup

⅛ teaspoon + ¹⁄₁₆ teaspoon sea salt

MINTY POMEGRANATE

2 cups brewed unsweetened mint tea, cooled

1 cup pomegranate juice

1 tablespoon fresh lemon juice

⅛ teaspoon + ¹⁄₁₆ teaspoon sea salt

Combine all of the ingredients for the flavor of your choosing in a water bottle and shake well.

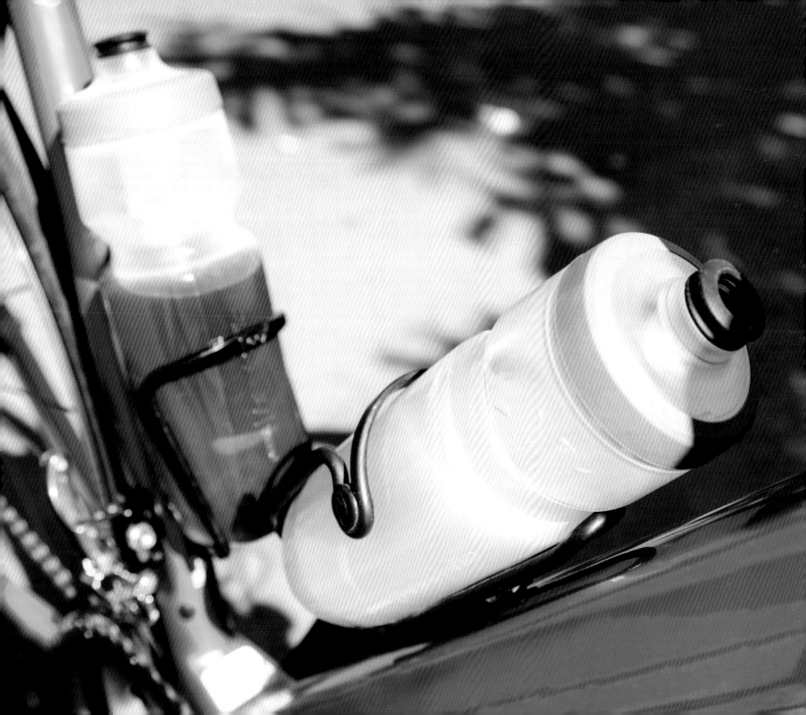

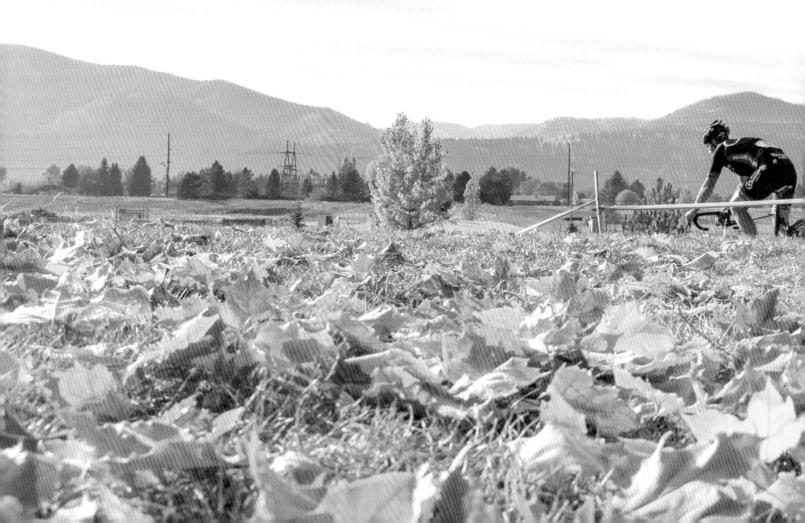

Good nutrition over the long haul is key to success.
In other words, think marathon, not sprint.

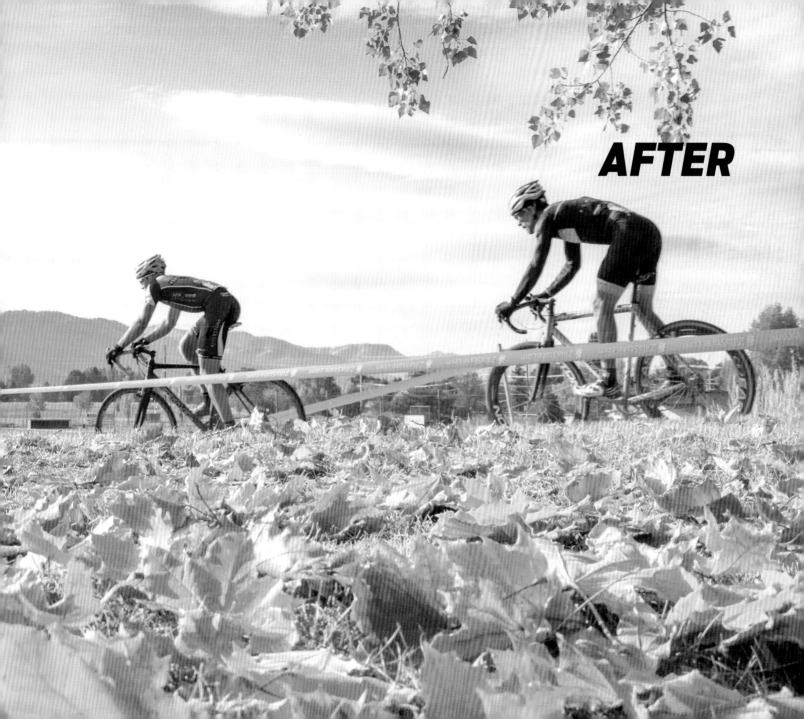

AFTER

RECHARGE AND RECOVER

AS THE OLD SAYING GOES, "Breakfast is the most important meal of the day." It's true that a well-balanced morning meal brings about a slew of benefits, including better concentration and less chance that the needle moves in the wrong direction when you step on the scale. Yet those who train hard understand that the path to improved fitness gains and sport performance becomes much smoother when post-workout nutrition is taken just as seriously as breakfast.

That's because the hour or so after working out is considered a key time frame for kick-starting the replenishment of spent energy stores and switching on the machinery that is involved in repairing and building muscle in response to the physiological stressor known as exercise. In other words, after a workout your weary muscles are primed for nourishment. So if you give little thought to your post-training nutrition, it should come as no surprise that your time in the weight room or on the trail is producing lackluster results and that you are unable to respond properly to increased training volume.

The upshot of all of this is that while your overall diet is still the most crucial element when it comes to recovering from regular training and obtaining more returns on any given time investment, what you eat after working up a sweat plays a necessary role in showing your muscles some love. And if more exercise is on tap in the near future, proper post-workout fueling becomes even more crucial. Trying to play nutritional catch-up later on is not conducive to peak performance. But refuel properly and you'll be ready to hit the gym floor, pavement, or dirt again with vigor to spare.

CARB UP

Some depletion of liver and muscle carbohydrate (i.e., glycogen stores) is inevitable during exercise, whether it's running, cycling, or weight training. And your body becomes much more dependent on glycogen and less reliant on fat at higher exercise intensities that hover over 75 percent of maximal effort compared to efforts below 60 percent of max output. So the more charged up a workout, the greater the toll it will take on your glycogen stores. Since glycogen is the most important fuel source for hard-charging muscles (roughly 1 to 2 percent of the weight of lean body mass can be glycogen), replacing these stores following exercise should be just as important as updating your Strava status. If you wait too long, glycogen replenishment can be compromised and you may fall flat during subsequent exercise. The cessation of exercise is such a great time to stock up on glycogen because that's when enzymes, particularly glycogen synthase, involved in converting sugars into glycogen as well as transporters that bring nutrients into muscle cells are particularly revved and ready to help replenish your spent energy stores. So it only makes sense to supply these enzymes and transporters with the raw goods needed to get the job done—namely, carbohydrates from food.

Taking the necessary dietary steps to restock your glycogen is especially important when taking part in repeated bouts of daily exercise. This was played out in a 2015 *Medicine and Science in Sports and Exercise* study that found that trained volunteers who completed an initial run to exhaustion at 70 percent of maximum effort followed by a 4-hour recovery period were able to run nearly twice as long until exhaustion during a second exercise session if they consumed a high-carb beverage at 30-minute intervals during recovery compared to a low-carbohydrate drink. The

CONSUME

1.25–1.5 GRAMS OF CARBS

PER KILOGRAM OF WEIGHT IN THE

FIRST HOUR

AFTER EXERCISE

POWER POWDERS

Not just for weight lifters, the various types of protein powders can be a convenient way to get the protein your body needs after a workout—and they're easier to swallow than chicken breast. Rich in all the essential amino acids—particularly leucine, the most anabolic of all amino acids—milk-derived whey protein has long been a gold-standard protein powder. Fast-digesting whey protein isolate is a very pure form of whey protein, so it contains very little if any carbs, fat, or lactose. Less expensive whey protein concentrate can contain a little less protein and more carbs (i.e., lactose) or more fat per gram of powder, but it is also up to the task of stimulating recovery.

You can even choose whey sourced from grass-fed cattle for a more planet-conscious (and animal welfare–conscious) choice. I most often turn to whey when I want to include a protein powder in a recipe such as Recovery Ice Cream (p. 216) without altering the overall flavor. Whey tends to have a more neutral flavor than many of its counterparts, such as egg, hemp, or pea protein.

Beyond whey, the market has swelled to include many other protein options. You can now enrich your post-training smoothies with egg white powder, beef protein powder (*gracias*, Paleo-ers), and an array of vegetarian options including hemp, rice, soy, and pea. Try to avoid powders that include cheap fillers and bulking agents such as cellulose.

Veg-heads should rejoice that science is starting to show that concentrated vegetarian protein powders can bring about similar improvements in muscle recovery as animal-based powders, along with a lower carbon impact and possibly less digestive woes for some people. To reduce my intake of added sugar, I most often select plain-flavored protein powder and simply add healthier flavoring options such as berries, raw cacao powder, or pure vanilla extract.

runners' muscle glycogen levels were higher at the end of the recovery period when the carb-rich beverage was consumed, and it gave them the extra energy reserves they needed to keep on moving.

The best way endurance athletes can replenish their liver and muscle glycogen stocks is to consume roughly 1.25 to 1.5 grams of carbohydrates per kilogram of body weight in the first hour or so following the cessation of exercise. That means that a 150-pound runner who just finished pounding the pavement for a couple hours can benefit from a refueling program that includes at least 85 to 100 grams of carbs. Wait too long, say about 2 hours or more, to take in carbohydrates and glycogen synthesis could be reduced by up to 50 percent, which sets the stage for poor performance during follow-up training.

PROTEIN PUMP

Since muscle fibers experience various degrees of damage (micro-tears) during exercise, the addition of protein to your post-exercise nutrition plan is necessary to rebuild the structural aspects of your muscle. Even endurance activities such as mountain biking and trail running can bring about various degrees of muscular damage, and the muscles need protein for repair.

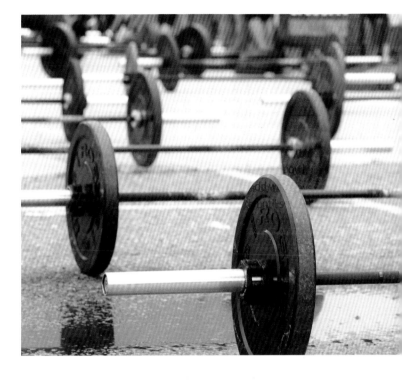

After exercise, when catabolic hormones are circulating at higher levels, the human body has a tendency to decrease its rate of protein synthesis (the process that takes protein from food and morphs it into muscle tissue) in favor of an increased rate of protein breakdown, which can heighten muscle soreness and possibly compromise training adaptations and subsequent performance. However, the provision of dietary protein (or, more accurately, the amino acids that make up protein) can reverse this trend, increasing protein synthesis and decreasing protein breakdown. You basically end up with more than you had when you started. This can inevitably lead to stronger, bigger, and more functional muscles, which not only make you look better but will also bring about noticeable strength, speed, and endurance improvements in your sport of choice via muscular remodeling. Consuming dietary protein after exercise is tantamount to providing a contractor with the bricks needed to rebuild your house into something bigger and better. Dietary protein can also help support an increase in mitochondrial protein, which produces muscles that are better at generating energy and are more resistant to fatigue during long runs, treks, and rides.

However, this doesn't mean you need to slice into Flintstone-sized steaks after working out. Recent research has found that just 20 grams of protein following resistance exercise is enough to speed muscle repair and growth. Although more protein won't do any harm, it will likely not provide any significant benefit to your muscles. Of course, protein should be consumed during other meals and snacks throughout the day to stay on top of whole-body muscle protein synthesis. In fact, a recent review of studies published in the *Journal of the International Society of Sports Nutrition* reported that consuming a protein-rich meal several hours after working out plays a big part in optimizing muscle gains. This demonstrates that the window of opportunity doesn't necessarily slam shut within an hour or so following exercise and is more proof that the nutrition segment of a training program extends to all waking hours.

DYNAMIC DUO

More proof that two heads are better than one: When carbohydrates and protein are combined in a snack or meal, there is a greater release of insulin than would occur if either was consumed alone. The hormone insulin functions to shuttle sugars and amino acids to muscle cells so they can be soaked up to set the stage for glycogen resynthesis and to encourage positive protein balance to allow for muscular repair and growth.

The stress that intense exercise places on your body also has a tendency to raise levels of cortisol, a stress hormone that can encourage increased muscle breakdown (bad if you're trying to get buff) as well as inflammation and immune suppression that can set you up for an illness

FOR ENDURANCE EXERCISE, USE A 4 TO 1 CARBS:PROTEIN RATIO FOR RECOVERY FUEL

that will leave you watching from the sidelines. But this doesn't mean you shouldn't give it your all during workouts; consuming the duo of carbohydrates and protein after exercise is an important part of preventing cortisol levels from spiking.

FOR **RESISTANCE TRAINING,** USE A **2 TO 1 CARBS:PROTEIN** RATIO FOR RECOVERY FUEL

Science still needs to pinpoint the exact ratio of carbs to protein that brings about optimal recovery, but individuals who just participated in endurance exercise such as running or road riding should seek out a ratio of about 4 to 1 to help replace spent carbohydrate stores and repair any muscular damage that occurred. If your workout of choice involved more resistance movements, such as weight training or CrossFit, you can bring the ratio closer together, say around 2 to 1, since carbohydrate stores will likely not have been as depleted but muscular stress can be significantly higher.

FAT CHANCE

Where does fat fit into the recovery plan? Although dietary fat is the least vital of the three macronutrients when it comes to recovery from exercise, it nonetheless has a role to play. First, it can contribute calories

FAST AND FURIOUS RECOVERY

Although I would never recommend a trip to the Golden Arches for your post-training fuel, an interesting report by researchers at the University of Montana helps once again illustrate that real food is just as good at promoting exercise recovery as what you might find in your local GNC. In the study, volunteers took part in two 90-minute bike rides designed to deplete their glycogen stores and then a 20K time trail after a 4-hour recovery period. During one recovery period, sports supplements such as bars and energy chews were provided. During the other recovery time frame, small portions of fast-food items, including burgers and fries, were consumed. Each provided the same number of calories, roughly 1,300. It turns out, rates of glycogen resynthesis from the feedings were the same, and there was no difference in time trial performance between the two diets. The takeaway is that recovery can be accelerated as long as the body is provided with the necessary amount of macronutrients, regardless of whether they come from tearing into engineered sports food or turning to food that requires a knife and fork. But for your overall health, you probably don't want fries with that.

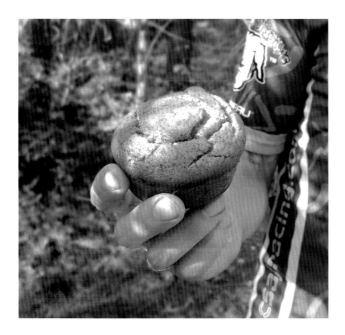

induced inflammation is less blood flow through the circulatory system, which in turn equates to fewer nutrients being delivered to muscle cells to instigate recovery from exercise.

Fat does, however, slow down transit through the digestive tract. So eating fat during the post-workout period may slow the digestion and absorption of carbohydrates and proteins. But studies have yet to prove that a reasonable amount of fat (read: not multiple slices of double-cheese pizza) in your post-training snack or meal can have a significant detrimental impact on the recovery process. That's why the post-training recipes that follow don't shy away from including moderate amounts of fat when needed. Besides, would you have bought this book if the post-training recipes were little more than sliced banana doused in whey protein?

LIQUID ASSETS

Beyond refueling and repairing, recovery nutrition should also include fluids and foods that promote rehydration and restoration of electrolyte balance. Monitoring the color of your urine is an easy way to gauge hydration status: Dark yellow pee and not needing to pee at all after a workout are good indications that it's time to have a drink. Athletes

(9 calories per gram) to an athlete's diet, which is particularly important when you're involved in a period of intense training where calorie needs are elevated. Fat also brings flavor, which can stimulate appetite— something that can wane after an intense bout of exercise—and thereby it allows a person to consume the necessary calories to support training. Healthy unsaturated fats from sources such as nuts, seeds, fatty fish, and avocado also work to reduce inflammation in the body. A potential side effect of increased exercise-

who want to be more precise with their post-training fluid needs can keep track of fluid losses by weighing themselves before and after training. For every pound of body weight lost, which is an indication of fluid lost, you should consume roughly 20 to 24 ounces of fluid. Fluids can come in the form of drinks but also from foods—namely fruits, which are made up of a large amount of water.

Moreover, electrolytes such as sodium and potassium found in various recovery foods and drinks will help replace what was lost in those beads of sweat. So while a high-sodium diet has been linked to health woes such as increased risk for stroke, if you just finished a sweatfest, you have permission to not shy away from sodium during your post-training fueling period (Yum, pretzels!). In fact, sodium can help with fluid retention to encourage better rehydration.

Of course, someone who spent several hours exercising in the great outdoors under a punishing sun will need to pay more attention to their post-training fluid and electrolyte needs than someone who spent 40 minutes on the elliptical machine in an air-conditioned fitness center.

CONSUME
20–24 OZ.
OF FLUID
FOR
EVERY
POUND
OF WEIGHT
LOST

However, a serious indoor interval workout such as a spinning session can cause a great deal of fluid and electrolyte loss via sweat, meaning that both of these aspects of recovery should be taken into account.

BATTLE OF THE BULGE

What is often overlooked is that post-exercise fueling may also help you maintain your race weight. How? Most sports nutritionists agree that you should supply your body with some nourishment within 1 hour after exercising. If you wait too long to eat after an 80-mile hammerfest, an overly spirited group run, or a tough CrossFit WOD, you may very well become hungry to the point where you turn into a ravenous cookie monster and end up overeating later on. By that time, the items you seek out to silence those hunger pangs may very well end up being nutritional duds like chips and candy that could lead to unwanted weight gain.

Save yourself from the desperation that leads to shoveling anything and everything edible into your mouth, regardless of its nutritional merits, or going to town at the nearest Taco Bell to help recoup spent calories. By embracing recipes that are specifically designed to refuel your body, you won't negate the efforts of your hard training.

READY-MADE RECOVERY

Following a hard workout, you can bounce back quicker by flooding your body with a mixture of carbohydrates, protein, antioxidants, and fluids to replace spent energy stores, jump-start muscle repair, and rehydrate.

The recipes in this chapter are my attempt to prove that recovery fuel need not be as boring as a packaged protein bar that's drier than the Sahara. In the pages that follow you'll find a collection of recipes that are not only what you need in order to recharge after training and get the results you want but that will also keep your taste buds happy. Many of the recipes aren't meant to be meals per se, but more along the lines of nutrient-dense post-training eats that have what it takes to get the recovery process moving along and to help tide you over until you can get a full-blown meal into your belly. Often, I'll combine two or more dishes, such as the Fruit and Grain Drink (p. 179) and Farro Egg Cakes (p. 195) or Chinese Pickled Eggs (p. 199) and Smoothie Cups (p. 170), to bolster carbohydrate and protein numbers to take the edge off my hunger.

Of course, the last thing you want to do immediately after stowing your bike, driving home from a trailhead, or shelving the dumbbells is to spend a bunch of time in the kitchen cooking up recovery fuel, especially if you're eager to get nourishment into your body lickety-split, as sports nutritionists encourage. That's why these recipes or elements of the recipes are designed so that they can be prepared ahead of time. Often nothing more is required on your part than quickly whirling something in a blender, boiling up some water, or slathering a spread on toast. It's the perfect way to end a workout on a high note.

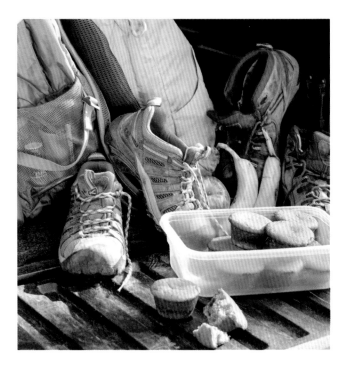

What I love most about having a jar of Instant Miso Noodle Soup (p. 196) or Chocolate Avocado Pudding (p. 219) ready to go is the anticipation factor. My final push on the bike always seems to be gutsier—yet seemingly less draining—if I know that I have something homemade and tasty waiting for me at the end of the ride. You don't want to find yourself staring into the fridge trying to figure out what to chow down on when you're suffering a case of exercise-induced brain fog.

Time to reinvent, recharge, and refresh!

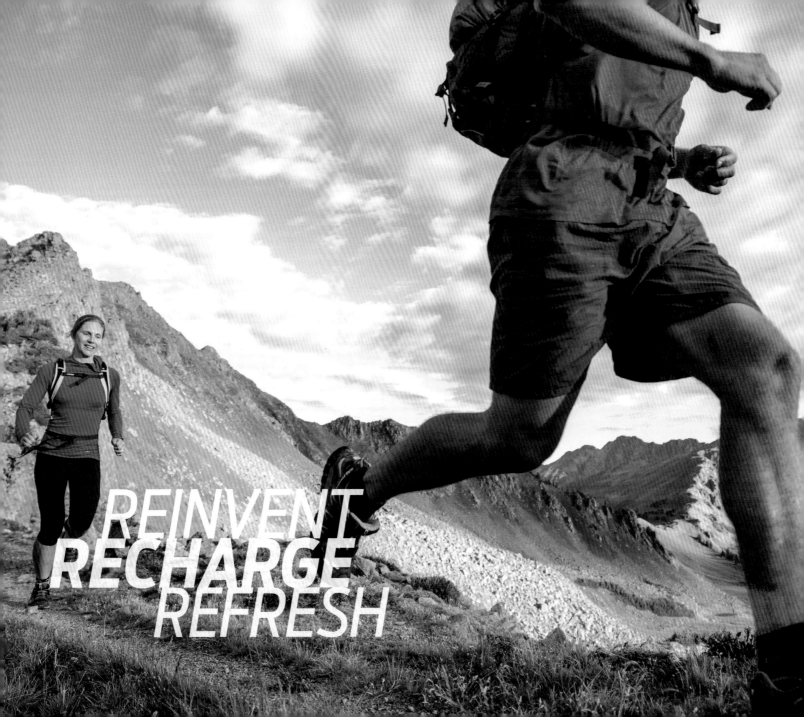

REINVENT
RECHARGE
REFRESH

RECIPES FOR **AFTER**

D **Dairy-free**   F **Freezer-friendly**   G **Gluten-free**   P **Paleo-friendly**   V **Vegetarian or vegan-friendly**

Look to the Game Changers section to find simple substitutions that make nearly every recipe more friendly for specific diets.

BLUEBERRY PROTEIN FREEZER PANCAKES

By thinking ahead and making up a batch of these protein-rich pancakes and freezing them, you can almost instantly enjoy a taste of breakfast for your recovery meal. Forget the fork and knife, just reheat and eat them hand-to-mouth style. Lemon zest adds a nice lemony essence to each bite.

D F G V

SERVINGS: 7
ACTIVE TIME: 20 min.

You can find cartons of ready-to-go egg whites in the egg section of most supermarkets. Since they're pasteurized, you can actually eat them straight from the container. Sometimes I even use leftovers to add a protein boost to my post-workout smoothies.

½ cup liquid egg whites or 4 regular egg whites
1 cup reduced-fat cottage cheese
1 medium-sized banana
¼ cup pure maple syrup
1½ cups oat flour
1 teaspoon cinnamon
1 teaspoon baking powder
½ teaspoon baking soda
Zest of 1 lemon
1 cup fresh or frozen blueberries

Place egg whites, cottage cheese, banana, maple syrup, oat flour, cinnamon, baking powder, baking soda, and lemon zest in a blender or food processor and blend until smooth. Stir in blueberries.

Lightly grease a large skillet or griddle with butter or cooking spray and heat over medium-low heat. Scoop ¼ cup batter for each pancake into pan and cook for 2 minutes per side, or until golden. Repeat with remaining batter, greasing pan as needed. You should end up with about 14 pancakes. Let pancakes cool completely on metal racks.

When cooled, place pancakes on a parchment paper–lined baking sheet and place tray in freezer until pancakes are completely frozen, about 4 hours. If space is tight, you can freeze pancakes in two batches. Once frozen, transfer pancakes to a zip-top freezer bag or other freezer-safe container and store frozen for up to 2 months.

To reheat, stack pancakes on a plate and microwave for 90 seconds, or until heated through. Or defrost and warm them using a toaster. You can also reheat in an oven or toaster oven set to 350°F.

GAME CHANGERS Use plain Greek yogurt or a dairy-free yogurt instead of cottage cheese + Go with spelt flour, whole wheat pastry flour, or a 1-to-1 gluten-free flour blend instead of oat flour

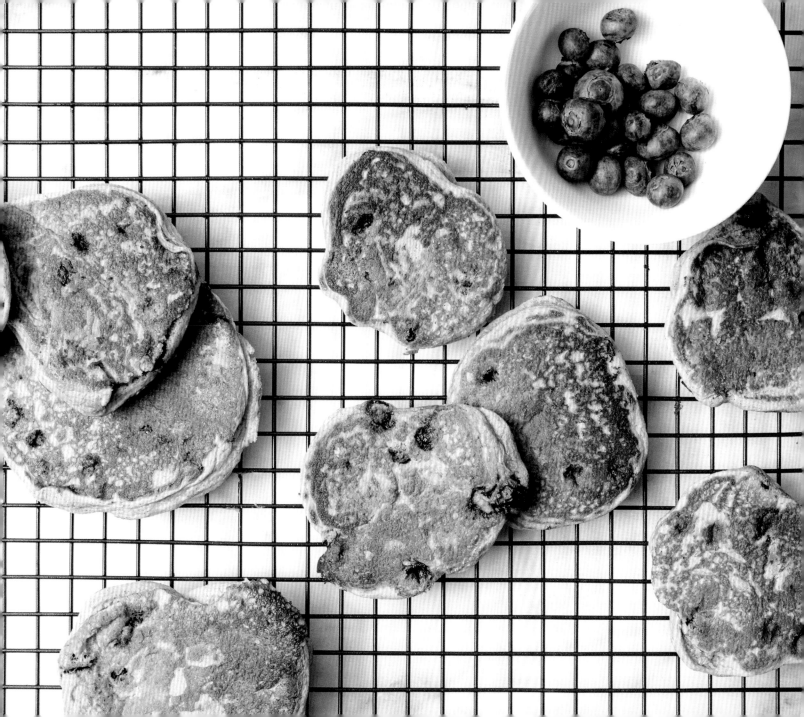

CANTALOUPE BOWLS WITH CRUNCHY QUINOA

These edible bowls are a refreshing way to wind down after a tough workout. Cantaloupe is an excellent hydrating fruit, while crispy cinnamon-scented quinoa provides a good textural contrast. And the bowls are stuffed with yogurt for a nice shot of muscle-building protein.

SERVINGS: 2
ACTIVE TIME: 10 min.

Beyond this recipe, crisp up any extra cooked quinoa you have on hand in the oven and sprinkle over vegetable or fruit salads and soups.

½ cup leftover cooked quinoa
1 teaspoon cinnamon
1 cup plain Greek yogurt
1 tablespoon honey
1 teaspoon vanilla extract
½ teaspoon ground ginger (optional)
1 cantaloupe

Preheat oven to 350°F. Stir together cooked quinoa and cinnamon. Place quinoa on a baking sheet lined with parchment paper or a silicone baking mat. Bake until crispy, 12 to 15 minutes, stirring once halfway through cooking. Remove from oven and let cool.

Stir together yogurt, honey, vanilla, and ground ginger, if using.

To serve, slice cantaloupe in half along its width, and then slice off about ½ inch from the bottoms of each melon half so they sit flat. Scoop out seeds and fill each melon half with yogurt mixture. Sprinkle on crispy quinoa.

GAME CHANGERS Swap out toasted quinoa for granola or muesli + Replace yogurt with cottage cheese, quark cheese, or dairy-free yogurt + Stir in maple syrup instead of honey + Use honeydew melon instead of cantaloupe

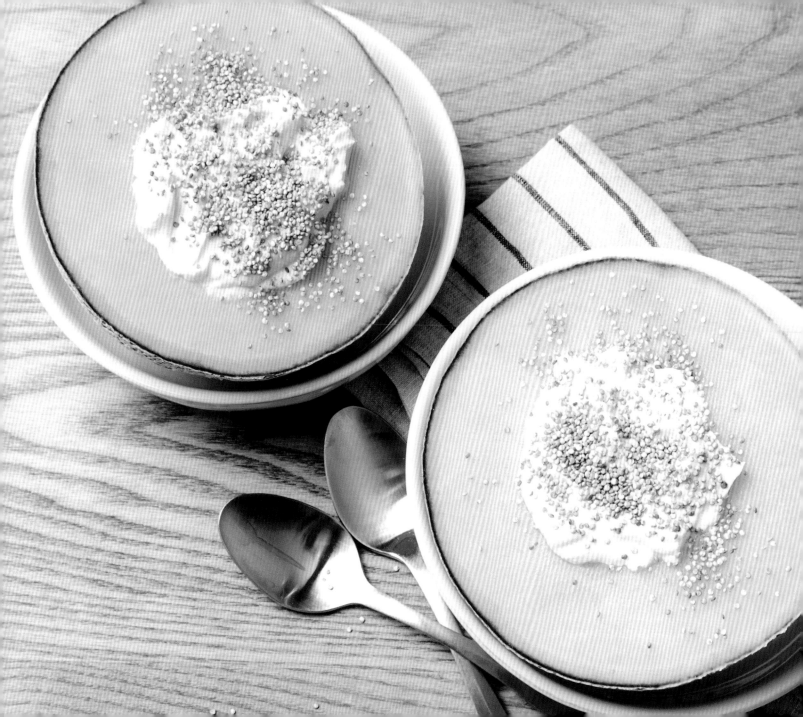

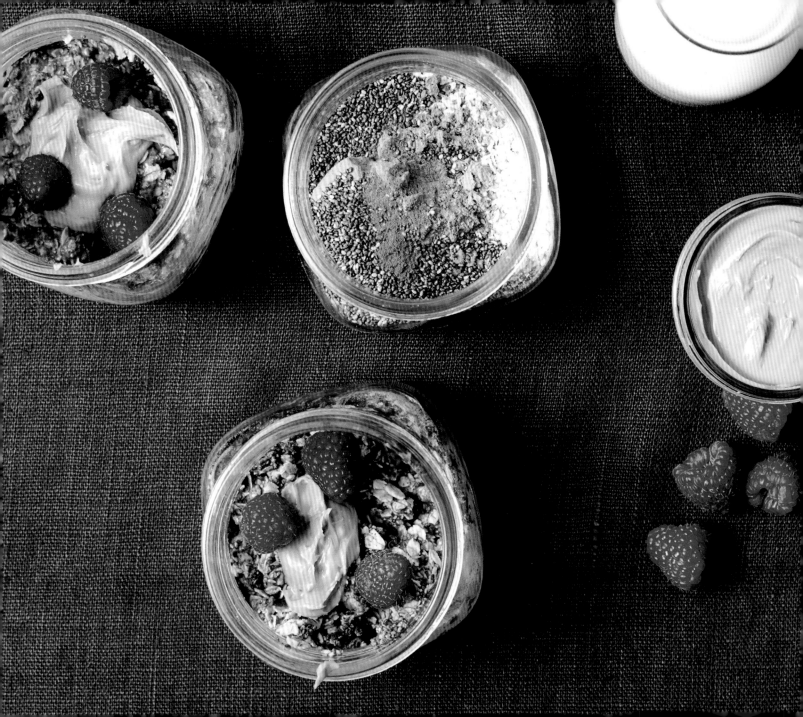

PB & BERRY PROTEIN OATS

More proof that breakfast is great at any time of day, these make-ahead gussied-up oats are ready to help you recover the minute your workout comes to a halt. Soaking the oats removes the need to cook them, making this recipe a great option for transporting with you if you're going to be away from the kitchen after exercise and you don't want to delay refueling.

SERVINGS: 1
ACTIVE TIME: 10 min.

Chia seeds are often added to overnight oat recipes since they do a great job of soaking up excess liquid to keep the mixture from being soggy.

½ cup rolled oats
¼ cup plain or vanilla protein powder
2 teaspoons chia seeds
¼ teaspoon cinnamon
⅔ cup low-fat milk
¼ teaspoon vanilla extract (optional)
1 tablespoon peanut butter
¼ cup fresh or frozen raspberries

In a wide-mouth half-pint glass jar, layer in oats, protein powder, chia seeds, and cinnamon. Stir in milk and vanilla if using. Top with peanut butter and raspberries. Seal shut and chill for 2 or more hours or up to 3 days.

GAME CHANGERS Use oats labeled "gluten-free" or try spelt, Kamut, or quinoa flakes instead of oats ✦ Replace protein powder with ¼ cup Greek yogurt and decrease milk to ½ cup ✦ To make dairy-free, use a plant-based protein powder and nondairy milk in place of milk ✦ Top with strawberries or blackberries instead of raspberries

CEREAL AND MILK

A bowl of cereal has long been athlete comfort food. And it turns out each spoonful can be recovery fuel, too. A *Journal of the International Society of Sports Nutrition* study found that a bowl of whole-grain cereal and milk was just as good at replenishing muscle-glycogen stores as a sports drink following 2 hours of moderate endurance exercise. It also did a better job at increasing protein synthesis, an indication of muscle repair. Why? Cereal and milk provide a dynamic duo of carbs and protein to promote recovery. Rather than settle for the standard stuff from a box, upgrade to this option featuring the gluten-free power grains amaranth and buckwheat along with antioxidant-laced tart cherries.

D G V

SERVINGS: 6
ACTIVE TIME: 20 min.

It can take a couple rounds to get the hang of popping amaranth, so keep some extra nearby if you end up singeing some. For added nutrition, top each bowl with fresh fruit such as berries or sliced banana.

½ cup uncooked amaranth
½ cup uncooked buckwheat groats
1 cup pecan halves
3 tablespoons pure maple syrup
2 teaspoons orange zest
½ teaspoon cinnamon
½ cup dried tart cherries
⅓ cup unsweetened flaked coconut
¼ cup cacao nibs
3 cups low-fat milk

Heat a medium-sized heavy-bottom saucepan over medium heat. When a drop of water energetically sizzles in the pan, add 1 tablespoon amaranth, cover pan with a lid, and shake the pan vigorously as soon as the grains begin to pop until most of the amaranth has popped. If amaranth burns, try shaking the pan about 1 inch above the burner when the popping begins. Remove popped amaranth from the pot and place in a large bowl. Repeat with remaining grain.

Heat a heavy skillet over medium heat. Add buckwheat groats and heat until darkened and fragrant, about 5 minutes, stirring often. Be careful not to burn the groats. Place groats in bowl with popped amaranth.

Add pecans, maple syrup, orange zest, and cinnamon to skillet. Heat 2 minutes, or until pecans are well glazed with syrup, stirring often. Place pecans on a baking sheet or cutting board to cool. Separate any pecans that have stuck together and place them in bowl with amaranth and groats. Stir in cherries, coconut, and cacao nibs. Store in an airtight container at room temperature for up to 1 week.

When ready to serve, place some cereal in a bowl and top with milk.

GAME CHANGERS Try dried blueberries or cranberries instead of cherries ✦ Replace cow milk with goat milk or nondairy milk

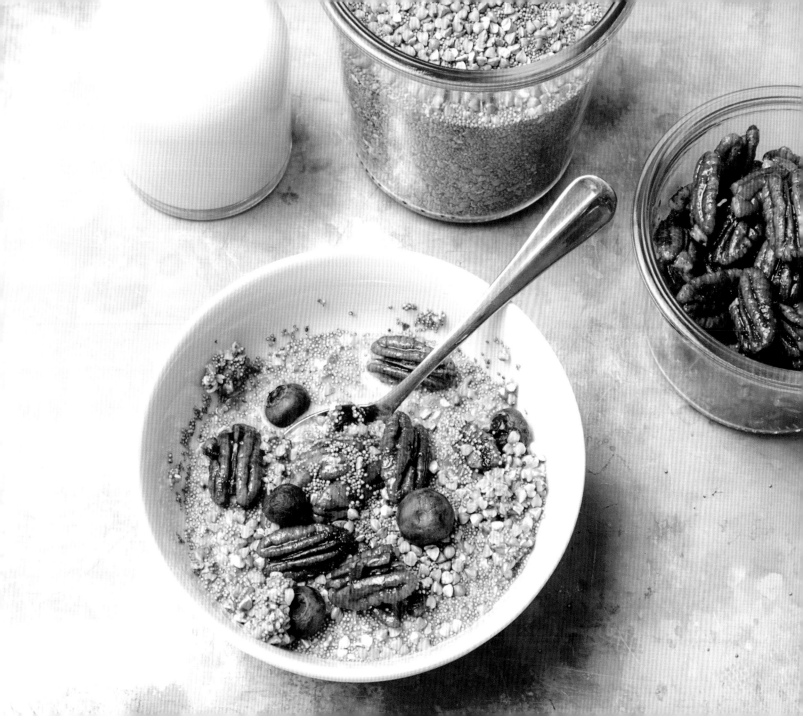

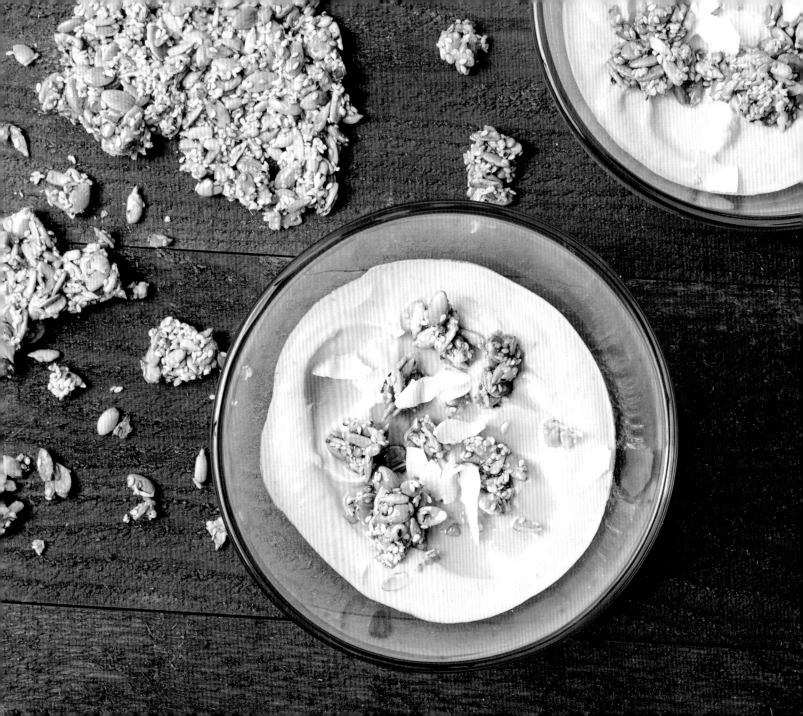

PUMPKIN PIE YOGURT BOWL
WITH SUPER SEED SPRINKLE

Deliciously thick Greek-style yogurt contains a wealth of protein to help guide your muscles on the path to recovery. Plus, it delivers probiotics for better immune and gut health. Stir in sweet pumpkin, maple syrup, and warming spices and then top it all off with nutrient-dense toasty seeds and you have a post-workout dish or mid-afternoon snack that tastes too sinful to be good for you.

G P V

SERVINGS: 4
ACTIVE TIME: 15 min.

Choose lower-fat varieties of Greek yogurt to keep your post-workout fat intake in check. My preference is 2% yogurt, which contains just enough fat to make it satiating.

Both the yogurt mixture and seeds can be prepared up to 5 days in advance but are best combined just before serving.

2 cups plain low-fat Greek yogurt
¾ cup canned pure pumpkin puree
¼ cup pure maple syrup, divided
1 teaspoon vanilla extract
½ teaspoon cinnamon
½ teaspoon ground ginger
¼ teaspoon ground cloves
¼ cup unsalted raw pumpkin seeds (pepitas)
¼ cup unsalted raw sunflower seeds
2 tablespoons sesame seeds
2 tablespoons hemp seeds
¼ cup unsweetened coconut flakes (optional)

Stir together yogurt, pumpkin, 2 tablespoons maple syrup, vanilla, cinnamon, ginger, and cloves. Chill until ready to use.

Heat a skillet over medium-low heat. Add pumpkin seeds and sunflower seeds and heat for 4 minutes, or until seeds are lightly golden, shaking the pan often. Add sesame seeds and heat until they are toasted, about 1 minute, stirring seeds often. Stir in hemp seeds, 2 tablespoons maple syrup, and a pinch of salt; heat 1 minute more. Spread out seed mixture on a baking sheet lined with parchment paper or a baking mat to cool. When cool, break up mixture into small chunks and store in an airtight container until ready to use.

To serve, place some yogurt in a serving bowl and top with seed mixture and coconut flakes if using.

GAME CHANGERS Replace spices with pumpkin pie spice ✦ Try cottage cheese instead of yogurt ✦ Swap out maple syrup for honey

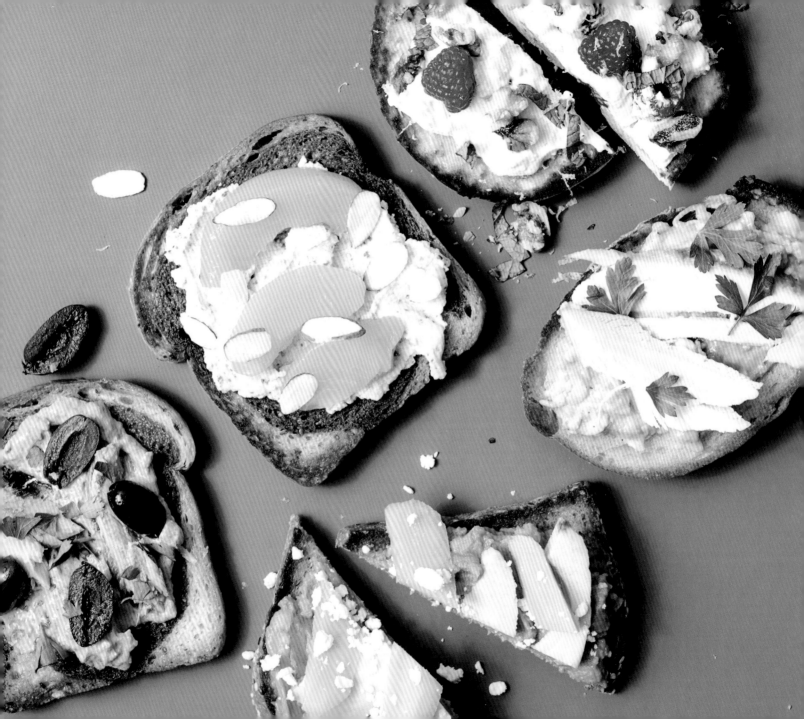

TOAST STACKS

No offense to peanut butter, but when it comes to recovery toast you can stack on a more inspiring combination of ingredients to deliver the carbs and protein you need to revive after a tough workout. Enjoy these even more by using crusty bread from a local artisanal baker. For an even bigger dose of recovery carbs, use a toasted bagel.

SERVINGS: 4
ACTIVE TIME: 5–10 min.

Beyond the toaster, crisp bread by placing a generous amount of olive oil (enough to cover the bottom of the pan) in a heavy skillet and turn the heat to medium-high. When the oil is hot, place the bread in the pan and heat until golden, 2 to 3 minutes per side. Or place oil-brushed bread slices directly on the grill and heat until grill marks appear, about 2 minutes per side.

4 thick slices of bread, toasted

GOING BANANAS
BASE
- 1 ripe avocado, mashed
- 1 small ripe banana, mashed
  Juice of ½ lime
- ¼ teaspoon chili powder
- ⅛ teaspoon salt

TOPPING
- 2 cups sliced roasted chicken
- ¼ cup cilantro

JUST PEACHY
BASE
- 1 cup reduced-fat ricotta cheese
- 2 tablespoons prepared pesto

TOPPING
- 2 peaches, sliced
- ¼ cup sliced almonds

COTTAGE COUNTRY
BASE
- 1 cup reduced-fat cottage cheese
- 1 cup fresh raspberries
- 2 teaspoons lemon zest

TOPPING
- ¼ cup chopped walnuts
- ¼ cup sliced fresh mint

GO FISH
BASE*
- ½ cup reduced-fat sour cream
- ½ cup peppadew peppers or roasted red pepper
- ⅓ cup oil-packed sun-dried tomatoes
- 1 garlic clove
- 1 tablespoon red wine vinegar
- ½ teaspoon fennel seeds (optional)
- ¼ teaspoon salt

* Combine ingredients in blender or food processor

TOPPING
- 2 (4.3-ounce) cans sardines packed in water
- ¼ cup sliced Kalamata olives
- ¼ cup chopped flat-leaf parsley

BEAN GOOD
BASE
- 1 cup fat-free refried beans

TOPPING
- 1 avocado, sliced
- 1 cup sliced mango
- 2 ounces diced feta cheese (about ½ cup)
  Squirt of lime juice

If your chosen flavor option's base has more than one ingredient, stir them together before applying. Apply an equal amount of a base and topping combo to each piece of toast.

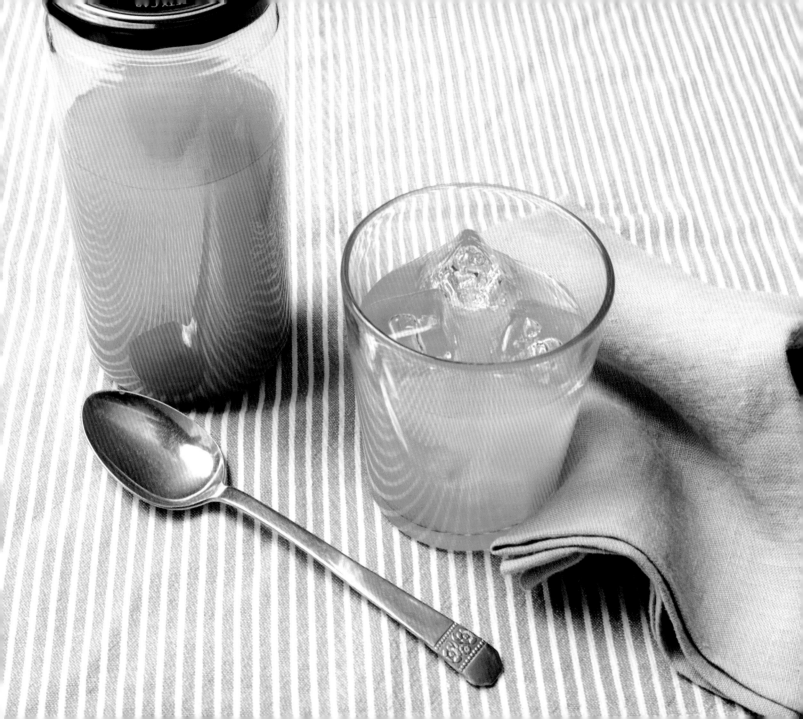

TURMERIC GINGER TONIC

More and more athletes are turning to turmeric and ginger for their anti-inflammatory powers. That makes this elixir a great way to simultaneously rehydrate and tame the flame. You can turn this into a warm drink for the cooler months by heating it on the stove top until hot to the touch, or it's a great hot summer night drink when mixed with club soda and served over ice.

SERVINGS: 4
ACTIVE TIME: 10 min.

I often freeze some fresh turmeric root, which makes it easier to grate when I want to use it to make a hot herbal tea.

3- to 4-inch piece fresh turmeric, thinly sliced
2-inch piece fresh ginger, thinly sliced
2 tablespoons honey
Juice of ½ orange

Place 4 cups water, turmeric, ginger, honey, and a pinch of salt in a medium saucepan. Bring to a boil, reduce heat to low, and simmer for 5 minutes. Remove from heat and let stand until cooled to room temperature. Stir in orange juice and then strain mixture into a glass jar. Chill until ready to serve, for up to 1 week. When ready to serve, place ice in a glass and pour in turmeric drink.

MELLOW YELLOW

Convert this into a post-training recovery shake by blending 1 cup turmeric drink with 1 cup chopped mango, 1 small chopped carrot, ⅓ cup plain or vanilla protein powder, and 1 small chopped frozen banana.

GAME CHANGERS Sweeten with agave syrup instead of honey + Use lime or lemon juice instead of orange

CHOCOLATE MILK

Studies show that guzzling chocolate milk after a stiff workout can improve muscle recovery and help you work harder during subsequent exercise. It has everything you need in one glass, namely the right combination of carbohydrates, protein, electrolytes, and fluid, which work synergistically to help you recharge. But homemade chocolate moo juice blows away anything from the grocery store. The syrup is also great on yogurt or ice cream. Consider whisking in about a teaspoon of instant espresso powder when making the syrup to perk it up. You can also mix it with milk that has been warmed in the microwave or on the stove top for a toasty drink when you've just finished up a workout in chilly temperatures.

SERVINGS: 4
ACTIVE TIME: 10 min.

For body-friendly antioxidants, use raw cocoa powder (often spelled *cacao*) instead of Dutch-processed, which is treated with alkali that destroys naturally occurring antioxidants. You can also up the nutritional ante by opting for organic or grass-fed milk, which has higher levels of beneficial nutrients such as omega fats.

⅓ cup brown sugar
⅓ cup unsweetened cocoa powder
1 teaspoon vanilla extract
4 cups low-fat milk

Combine the sugar and ⅓ cup water in a small saucepan. Bring to a simmer over medium heat. Whisk in the cocoa powder until smooth and no clumps remain, stirring constantly to prevent burning. Remove from the heat and stir in the vanilla. The mixture will be fairly thick. Let cool to room temperature before storing in the refrigerator for up to 2 weeks.

When ready to serve, place about 1 tablespoon chocolate syrup and a pinch of salt in a glass. Top with 1 cup milk and stir well until syrup has dissolved.

GAME CHANGERS Replace brown sugar with turbinado sugar, coconut sugar, or maple sugar + Replace cow milk with goat milk or plain or vanilla nondairy milk

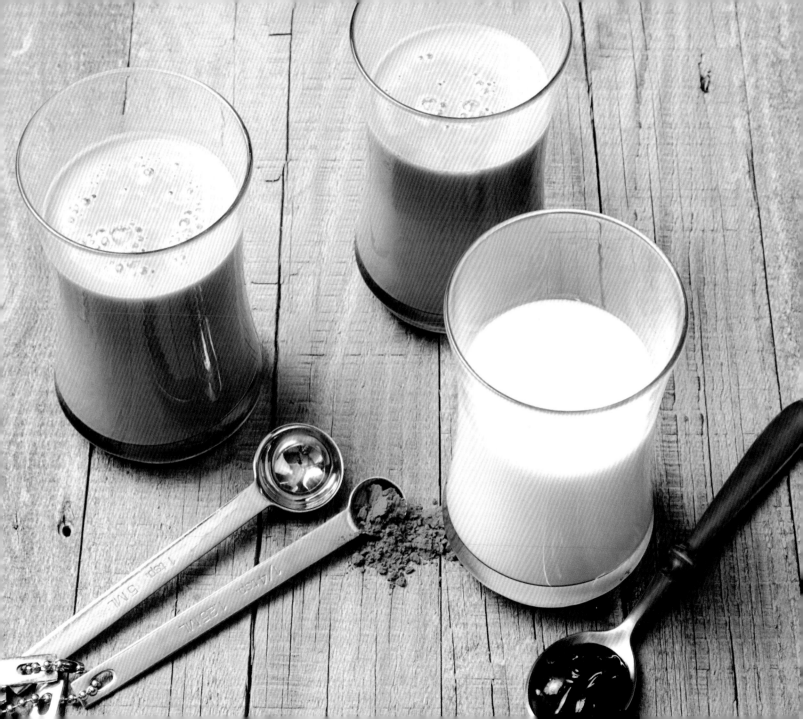

SMOOTHIE CUPS

Smoothies are an ideal way to quickly flood your body with recovery nutrients after a workout. Plus, they're easy to consume for those whose appetites wane after hard training. But gathering up all the necessary ingredients when you're zapped of energy can be a pain. That's why ready-to-whirl Smoothie Cups are your answer for a quick, frosty drink when you need it most. Simply drop a couple of the concentrated frozen cups into a blender with some additional liquid and you're good to go. For higher protein numbers, you can also blend in some extra protein powder.

D F G P V

SERVINGS: 6
ACTIVE TIME: 15 min.

Nonstick and bendable (read: easy extraction) silicone muffin cups are the way to go when it comes to making these subzero heroes.

THAI MANGO TANGO

- 1 cup coconut milk beverage
- 1 package (12 ounces) soft (silken) tofu
- 2 mangos, peeled and sliced
- 2 tablespoons peanut butter
- ⅓ cup fresh mint
- 2 tablespoons honey
- Zest of 1 lime
- Juice of 1 lime
- 1-inch piece fresh ginger, peeled
- ⅛ teaspoon chili powder

GREEN MONSTER

- 1 cup coconut water or tap water
- 1½ cups plain Greek yogurt
- 2 avocados, peeled and pits removed
- 2 seedless oranges, peeled and quartered
- 2 cups spinach
- ⅓ cup fresh basil
- 2 tablespoons honey
- 1-inch piece fresh ginger, peeled

MOCHA MADNESS

- 2 cups strongly brewed coffee, cooled to room temperature
- 3 medium-sized ripe bananas
- ½ cup protein powder
- ⅓ cup hazelnuts
- ¼ cup unsweetened cocoa powder
- ¼ cup unsweetened shredded coconut
- 2 teaspoons vanilla extract
- ¾ teaspoon cardamom powder

CHERRY CHEESECAKE

- 1 cup plain almond milk
- 1½ cups part-skim ricotta cheese
- 2 cups pitted fresh or frozen cherries
- ¼ cup hemp seeds
- ¼ cup fresh mint
- Zest of 1 lemon
- 1 teaspoon almond extract (optional)
- 1 teaspoon cinnamon

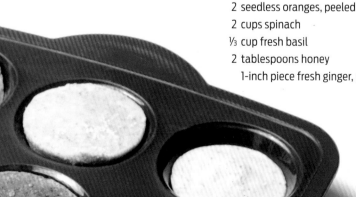

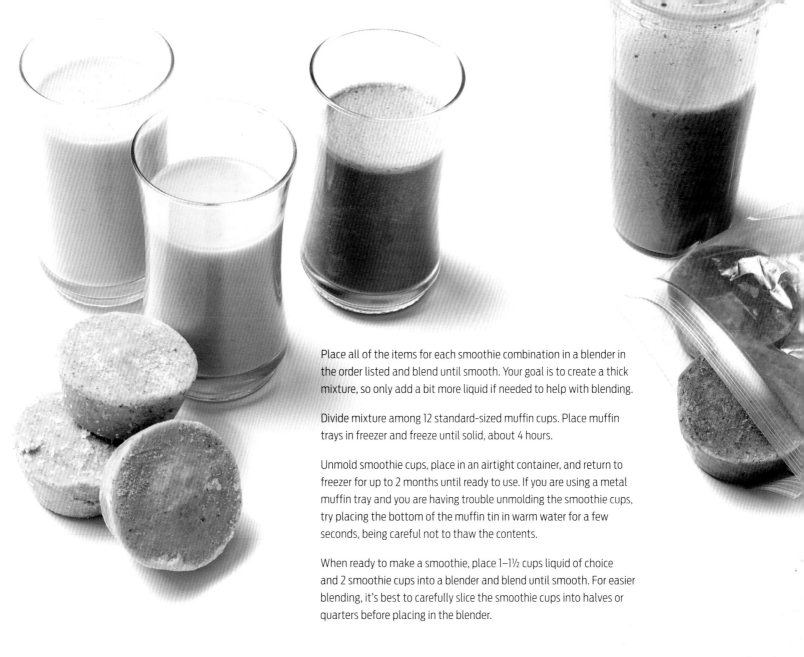

Place all of the items for each smoothie combination in a blender in the order listed and blend until smooth. Your goal is to create a thick mixture, so only add a bit more liquid if needed to help with blending.

Divide mixture among 12 standard-sized muffin cups. Place muffin trays in freezer and freeze until solid, about 4 hours.

Unmold smoothie cups, place in an airtight container, and return to freezer for up to 2 months until ready to use. If you are using a metal muffin tray and you are having trouble unmolding the smoothie cups, try placing the bottom of the muffin tin in warm water for a few seconds, being careful not to thaw the contents.

When ready to make a smoothie, place 1–1½ cups liquid of choice and 2 smoothie cups into a blender and blend until smooth. For easier blending, it's best to carefully slice the smoothie cups into halves or quarters before placing in the blender.

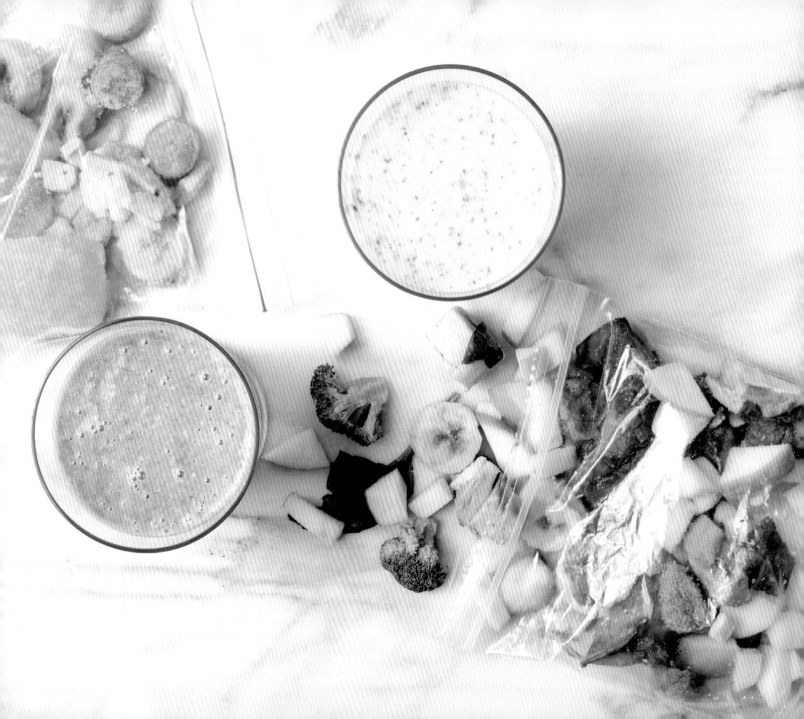

SMOOTHIE PACKS

Similar to Smoothie Cups, these ready-when-you-are frozen packs are a superb way to enjoy a nutrient-dense icy-cold recovery drink quickly after a workout, but without the need for pre-blending and freezing in muffin cups. They're also great for mornings when you only have a moment to breathe. Simply place the main players in freezer bags and then blend with a couple of add-ins.

SERVINGS: 4
ACTIVE TIME: 15 min.

If the contents of the bag freeze together, be sure to break them apart first by hitting the bag against the counter before adding to blender. This is especially important if you don't have a machine with big-time horsepower.

ORANGE CRUSH

FROZEN ITEMS

2 medium-sized carrots, roughly chopped
2 oranges, peeled and quartered
  2-inch piece fresh ginger, peeled and roughly chopped
2 medium-sized bananas, peeled and roughly chopped

ADD-INS

6 cups coconut water or tap water
1 cup plain or vanilla protein powder
8 teaspoons tahini
1 teaspoon ground allspice

Divide frozen items among 4 zip-top bags, press out as much air as possible, and freeze for up to 3 months.

When ready for a smoothie, place 1½ cups liquid, ¼ cup protein powder, 2 teaspoons tahini, ¼ teaspoon ground allspice, and the contents of 1 bag in a blender and blend until smooth.

GREEN POWER

FROZEN ITEMS

2 avocados, peeled and cubed
4 cups spinach
2 cups broccoli florets
½ cup fresh mint leaves
  2-inch piece fresh ginger, peeled and roughly chopped
2 green apples, chopped
2 medium-sized bananas, peeled and roughly chopped

ADD-INS

6 cups coconut water or tap water
2 cups plain yogurt
¼ cup fresh lemon juice

Divide frozen items among 4 zip-top bags, press out as much air as possible, and freeze for up to 3 months.

When ready for a smoothie, place 1½ cups coconut water, ½ cup yogurt, 1 tablespoon lemon juice, and contents of 1 bag in a blender and blend until smooth.

HOT CHOCOLATE RECOVERY SMOOTHIE

After a crisp late-fall run or a full day of cross-country skiing, you're not likely to be craving a frosty drink. That's the beauty of this smoothie: It's reminiscent of hot chocolate but with the carbs and protein needed for recovery.

SERVINGS: 1
ACTIVE TIME: 5 min.

If drinking right away, don't let the water come to a full boil or you'll need to wait several minutes until it's cool enough to drink. But if storing in an insulated container to drink later on, you can use boiling water to help the drink stay warmer for longer.

1½ cups water
¼ cup milk powder
1 small banana
1 tablespoon unsweetened cocoa powder
1 scoop protein powder of choice
2 teaspoons almond butter or other nut butter
½ teaspoon vanilla extract or peppermint extract
¼ teaspoon cinnamon
  Pinch of chili powder or cayenne powder (optional)

Heat water in a kettle to desired temperature. Place water in a blender along with remaining ingredients and blend until smooth. Consume immediately or transfer to an insulated drink container to keep warm until after your workout.

GAME CHANGERS Perk it up by replacing half of the water with hot brewed coffee ✦ Swap out milk powder for coconut milk powder ✦ Instead of a banana, blend in ½ avocado ✦ Add allspice instead of cinnamon

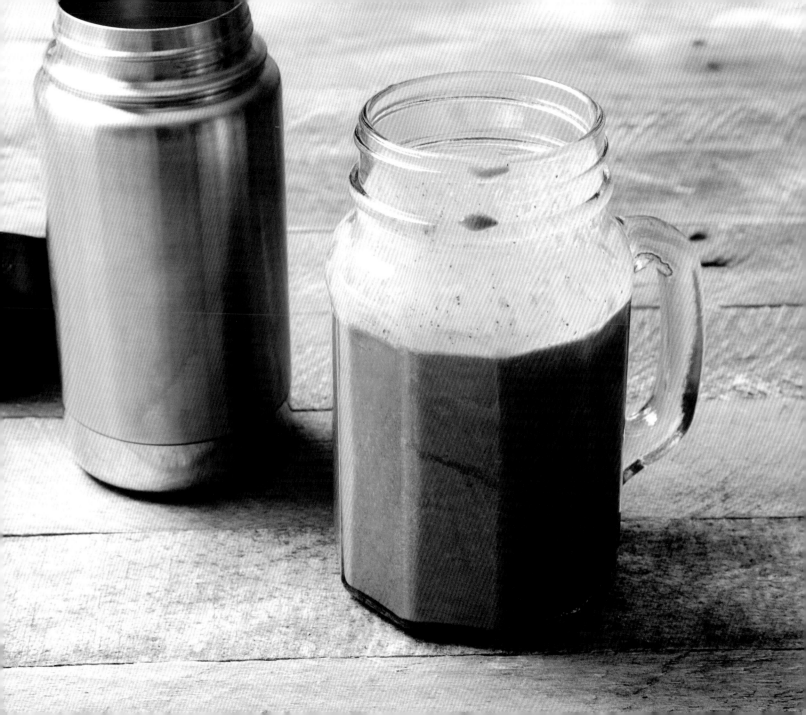

SWEET POTATO SHAKE

This rich and creamy drink is sure to shake up your recovery routine. Tangy kefir delivers protein and an even bigger dose of probiotics than yogurt. Recent research suggests that the friendly critters in fermented foods such as kefir can bolster immune health in athletes. Look for kefir in the dairy section alongside yogurt.

SERVINGS: 1
ACTIVE TIME: 10 min.

Packed with natural sweetness, sweet potato is one of the most overlooked smoothie ingredients, partly because of prep time. To help this shake go from blender to belly quickly, cook up a bunch of sweet potatoes all at once and then keep the cooked spuds chilled in the refrigerator for up to 5 days.

1 cup plain kefir
1 cup peeled and cubed sweet potato, cooked and cooled
1 scoop plain or vanilla protein powder (optional)
2 teaspoons almond butter
2 teaspoons pure maple syrup
½ teaspoon vanilla extract
¼ teaspoon cinnamon
¼ teaspoon ground ginger
⅛ teaspoon nutmeg
1 small frozen banana, chopped

Place all of the ingredients in a blender in the order listed and blend until smooth.

GAME CHANGERS Replace kefir with ½ cup Greek yogurt and ½ cup low-fat milk ✦ Whiz in cooked butternut squash instead of sweet potato ✦ Use peanut butter or cashew butter in place of almond butter ✦ Go with molasses over maple syrup

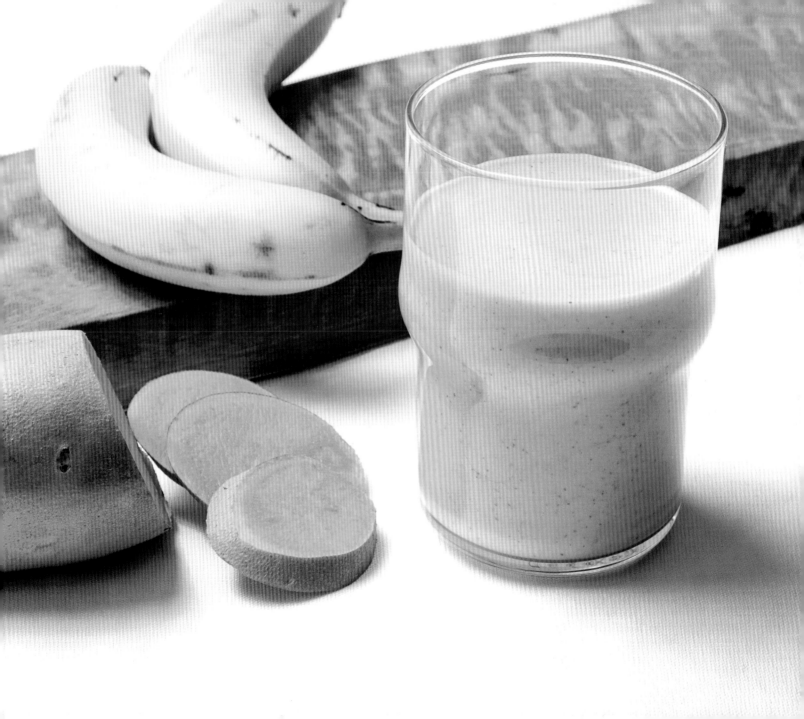

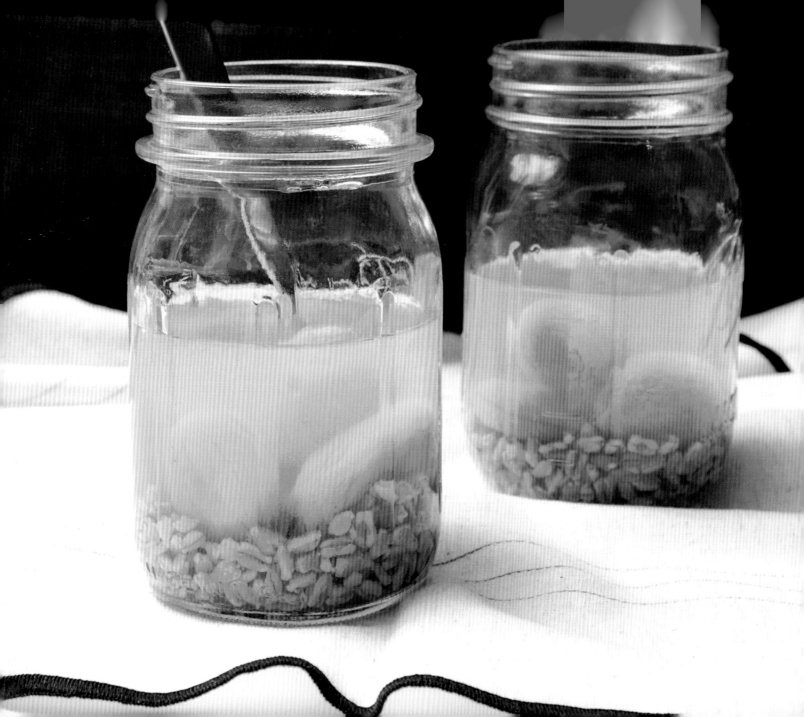

FRUIT AND GRAIN DRINK

Beyond the incredible volcanic scenery and cheap wine, what I remember most about cycling in Chile is *mote con huesillo*, a common drink consisting of cooked husked wheat (*mote*), sweet liquid syrup, and dried peaches (*huesillo*). It's a refreshing way to rehydrate and restock spent carbohydrate stores, and it can taste like an elixir from the gods after a hot sufferfest. For a different flavor, omit the ginger, cinnamon, and lemon juice, add 2 tablespoons orange pekoe loose-leaf tea to the warm water-honey mixture, and let cool. Strain out tea.

SERVINGS: 4
ACTIVE TIME: 10 min.

The chewy ancient grain spelt is a great alternative to husked wheat. It can take up 50 minutes to cook, so consider making a big batch and using extras in salads and soups. Or freeze cooked spelt for future batches of this recipe. Soaking spelt overnight before cooking can slash the cooking time by about 30 percent.

16 dried apricots (about ½ cup)
¼ cup honey
   1-inch piece fresh ginger, peeled and thinly sliced
1 cinnamon stick (optional)
   Juice of ½ lemon
1 cup cooked spelt

Place apricots and 6 cups water in a large container and let soak overnight or for several hours.

Drain apricots, saving the soaking liquid, and add the liquid to a medium-sized saucepan along with honey, ginger, and cinnamon stick, if using. Bring to a boil and simmer over medium-low heat for 10 minutes. Remove from heat and stir in lemon juice. Let cool to room temperature and then strain out solids. Return liquid to container with apricots and chill in the refrigerator for up to 10 days.

When ready to serve, place ¼ cup cooked spelt in the bottom of a wide-mouth glass jar and top with 4 apricots and about 1 cup honey liquid. Drinks can also be pre-assembled in jars and chilled for up to 5 days.

GAME CHANGERS If available, use dried peaches instead of apricots ✦ Sweeten liquid with agave syrup instead of honey ✦ Replace the spelt with farro, barley, wheat berries, or, for gluten-free, sorghum or millet

UMAMI TOMATO JUICE

Not just for cocktails, tomato juice is also a recovery aid. Studies have shown that the veggie-laden drink can help lessen oxidative stress, inflammation, and muscle damage in athletes after intense exercise. That all equals better recovery and potentially better performance. These benefits are likely owing to the blend of antioxidants in each sip. The addition of miso adds some umami savoriness along with beneficial probiotics.

SERVINGS: 4
ACTIVE TIME: 15 min.

To help improve the absorption of tomato juice's fat-soluble antioxidants such as lycopene, pair this drink with another recovery aid that contains a bit of fat such as the Edamame Hummus Wraps (p. 187).

1 cup water
3 medium tomatoes, quartered
2 celery stalks, sliced
1 red bell pepper, chopped
1 medium carrot, chopped
2–3 radishes, chopped (optional)
½ small yellow onion, diced
⅓ cup flat-leaf parsley
2–3 tablespoons white or yellow miso paste
1 garlic clove, chopped
Juice of ½ lemon
A few dashes hot sauce such as Tabasco or sriracha (optional)

Place all of the ingredients in a blender or food processor and blend until smooth, about 1 minute. If your container is small, you can do this in two batches. Place juice in a large glass container and chill in the refrigerator for at least 2 hours before serving or up to 5 days. Stir juice before serving as some separation will occur. If you want a thinner consistency, you can stir with some additional water prior to serving.

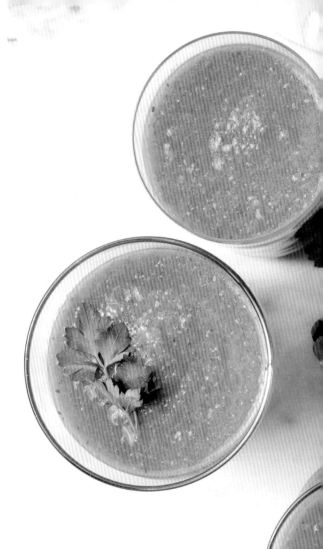

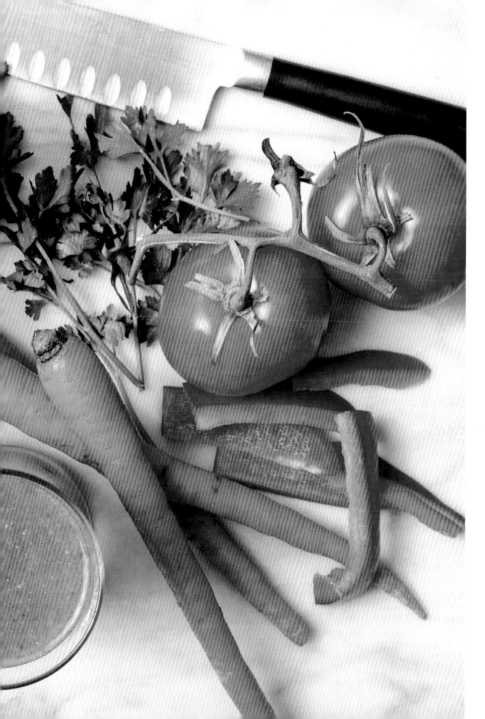

RED RIOT

Turn this juice into a recovery smoothie by blending together 1 cup Umami Tomato Juice, 1 cup frozen sweet cherries, ½ cup yogurt, ¼ cup fresh mint (optional), and 2 teaspoons honey until smooth.

BOTTOMS UP

Reward a job well done by serving up the Mexican beer cocktail *cerveza preparada*. Place a couple of ice cubes in a pint glass (salt the rim if you like) and top with equal amounts of tomato juice and light beer, preferably Mexican. Stir in juice of ½ lime and a couple dashes of Worcestershire sauce and hot sauce.

BLOODY MARY

Mix with an ounce of vodka and a few dashes of cayenne and/or Worcestershire sauce and serve over ice.

GAME CHANGERS For a little extra kick, use peppadew peppers instead of red bell pepper **+** Replace the onion with two sliced scallions (green onions) **+** Use fresh basil instead of parsley

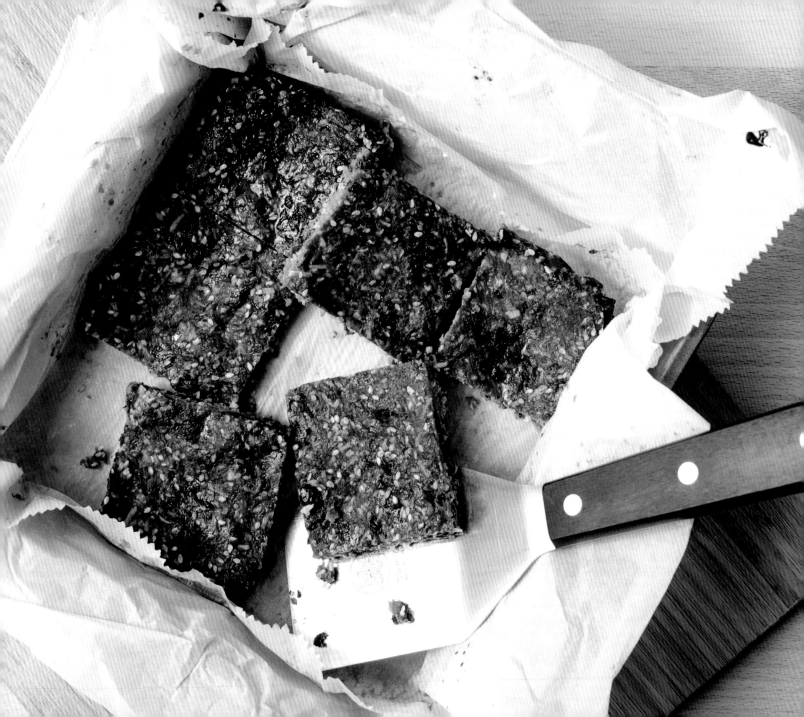

BEAST BARS

Time to unleash your inner Arrr! Jerky–energy bar hybrids are at the forefront of the energy bar revolution. Consider this tender and protein-packed DIY version your tribute to the mammoth-hunting caveman of yesteryear. Each bar also supplies a shot of energy-boosting iron, particularly important for active women.

 There are two important ingredients that keep these bars from tasting like leftover meatloaf. First, the cranberries offer up some of the sweetness that you would expect in a bar. And round steak, one of the leanest cuts available, is used to keep the fat levels low and help the mixture dry out in the oven. Too much fat will encourage the bars to go rancid more quickly. A longer cooking time at a low temp helps with the drying process.

D **G** **P**

SERVINGS: 9
ACTIVE TIME: 20 min.

Consider opting for grass-fed or organic beef. Studies suggest that steaks from grass-fed cattle are more nutrient dense than those from their grain-fed brethren, while organic beef is not administered hormones or antibiotics.

- 10 ounces round steak (eye, top, or bottom cut)
- 1 cup dried cranberries
- ¼ cup soy sauce
- ¼ cup unsweetened shredded coconut
- 3 tablespoons sesame seeds
- 2 teaspoons orange zest
- ½ teaspoon salt

Trim any excess fat from meat and cut into 1-inch cubes. Place on a parchment paper–lined baking sheet and freeze until edges are stiff but not frozen all the way through, about 20 minutes. This will help the meat grind more uniformly.

Preheat oven to 225ºF. Place partially frozen meat and cranberries in a food processor and pulse until meat is coarsely ground. Pulse in remaining ingredients.

Line an 8 × 8–inch square baking pan with a piece of parchment paper large enough so there is a 1-inch overhang. Place meat mixture in pan and spread out into an even layer. Bake for 30 minutes, pour off any accumulated juices, and then bake for another 50 minutes. Let cool completely in pan before lifting out with parchment overhang and cutting into 9 bars. Keep chilled for up to 1 week.

GAME CHANGERS Try dried cherries instead of cranberries + Use liquid aminos or gluten-free soy sauce instead of regular soy sauce + Replace sesame seeds with hemp seeds + Swap out the orange zest for lemon zest

TUNA BALLS

These little balls of protein and carbs are the ultimate in fanciful post-training food. Bring them to feed an active crowd and they are sure to disappear quickly. Research suggests that curcumin, the phytochemical that gives curry powder its yellow hue, may help reduce inflammation and muscle soreness in response to strenuous exercise. These are great straight from the fridge or cooler, but you can also warm them in the microwave.

D F G P

SERVINGS: 8
ACTIVE TIME: 20 min.

Canned tuna can be sketchy with respect to sustainability and contaminants. Your best defense? Splurge for cans from smaller-scale companies such as Wild Planet or Raincoast Trading. They employ less-destructive fishing methods and pack in more nutrient-dense (and more delicious!) tuna that is lower in contaminants such as mercury.

⅔ pound potato (about 1 medium-sized), peeled and cubed
2 (5-ounce) cans water-packed albacore or skipjack tuna, drained and flaked
1 large egg, lightly beaten
¼ cup golden raisins
2 tablespoons tahini
¼ cup finely chopped flat-leaf parsley
1 scallion (green onion), chopped
Juice of ½ lemon
1½ teaspoons yellow curry powder
½ teaspoon salt
¼ teaspoon black pepper

Steam or boil potato until tender.

Preheat oven to 350°F. Place potato in a large bowl and mash. Stir in remaining ingredients. Form into balls slightly smaller than golf ball–sized. You should have about 16 balls. Arrange on a lightly greased or parchment paper–lined baking sheet and bake for 35 to 40 minutes, or until darkened and crispy on the outside. Let cool and then store in an airtight container in the refrigerator for up to 5 days.

GAME CHANGERS Try canned salmon in place of tuna + Add chopped dried apricots in lieu of golden raisins + Mix in chopped basil instead of parsley

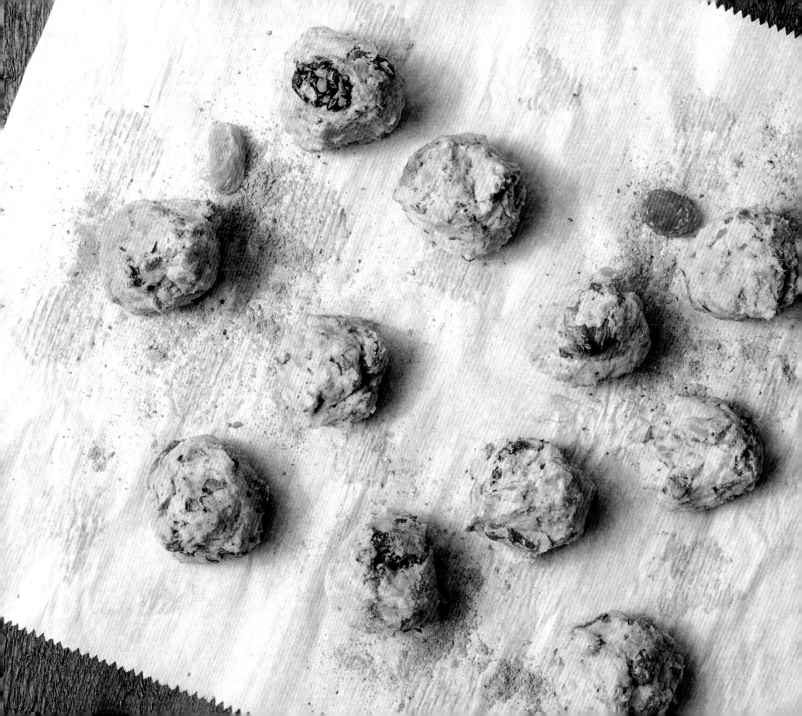

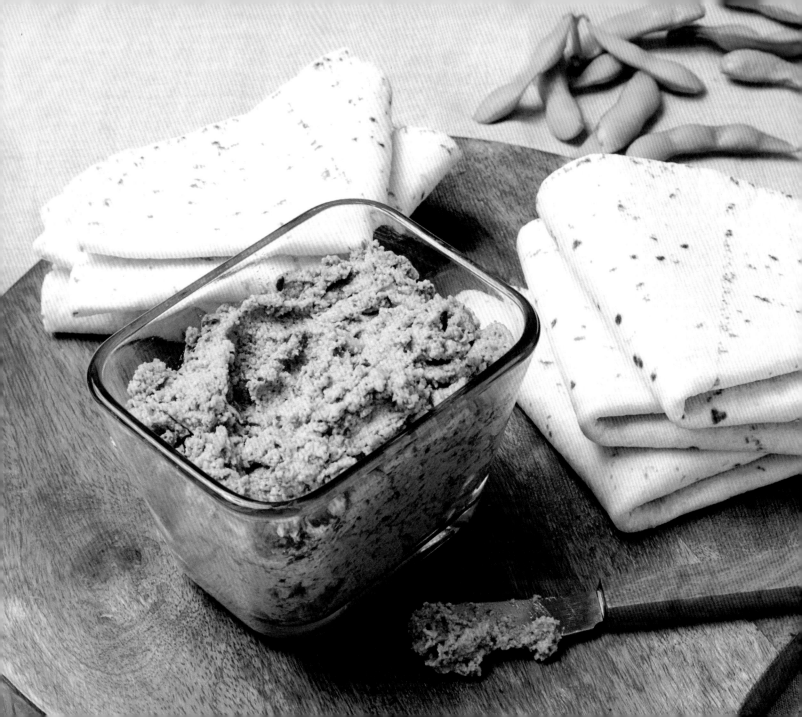

EDAMAME HUMMUS WRAPS

It can be a delicious diversion to think beyond smoothies for your post-training protein fix. Edamame, green soybeans found in the frozen vegetable section of grocers, pack in about 8 grams of protein per half-cup serving, along with an alphabet of vitamins and minerals, including folate, iron, and vitamin C. They serve as a nutritious alternative to chickpeas in this verdant hummus that gets wrapped up in a tortilla to help replenish those spent carbohydrate stores.

D F G V

SERVINGS: 6
ACTIVE TIME: 15 min.

Turn this into a healthy lunch by layering on sliced veggies such as carrot, red bell pepper, and cucumber, and even proteins such as roasted chicken, smoked tofu, or canned tuna.

2 cups frozen shelled edamame
2 cups spinach, stems trimmed
⅓ cup fresh mint
¼ cup tahini
2 tablespoons extra-virgin olive oil
1 garlic clove, minced
   Juice of 1 lemon
½ teaspoon cumin powder
½ teaspoon salt
¼ teaspoon chili powder
6 tortillas

Prepare edamame according to package directions. Drain well and let cool.

Place all of the ingredients except the tortillas in a food processor and blend until smooth. Chill edamame hummus for up to 5 days and freeze extras for up to 2 months. To serve, spread some of the edamame hummus on a tortilla and roll.

GAME CHANGERS Swap out spinach for Swiss chard + Use basil instead of mint + Replace the tortillas with rice cakes or gluten-free tortillas

APRICOT GRILLED CHEESE

While everyone seems to be ganging up on gluten these days, most athletes need not shelve their bread. A 2015 Australian study found that following a gluten-free diet provided no performance or digestive health benefits for nonceliac athletes. But of course if you really can't or don't want to eat gluten, there are a lot of decent gluten-free breads available. No one should have to give up hot, gooey grilled cheese. It's a blissful way to get your recovery carbs and protein.

SERVINGS: 6
ACTIVE TIME: 10 min.

A cast-iron skillet is made for producing great grilled cheese, as the heavy metal turns out deliciously toasted bread—just another reason to add ye olde iron skillet to your kitchen arsenal.

  1 cup dried apricots
  1 teaspoon dried thyme
12 slices bread
  6 ounces Brie cheese
  3 cups fresh spinach
  1 tablespoon butter

Place apricots, thyme, and 1¼ cups water in a glass container. Seal shut and let soak overnight.

Add apricots, remaining soaking liquid, and a pinch of salt to a blender or food processor and blend into a slightly chunky mixture. Add additional water, 1 tablespoon at a time, if needed to help with blending.

To make each grilled cheese, spread a generous amount of apricot jam on a slice of bread. Top with 1 ounce Brie cheese, a handful of greens, and another slice of bread. Heat butter in a skillet over medium heat. Cook sandwich until cheese is melted and bread is golden brown, about 2 minutes per side.

GAME CHANGERS Replace apricot spread with slices of fresh peaches ✦ Use gluten-free bread ✦ Swap out Brie cheese for mozzarella ✦ Use arugula or Swiss chard instead of spinach

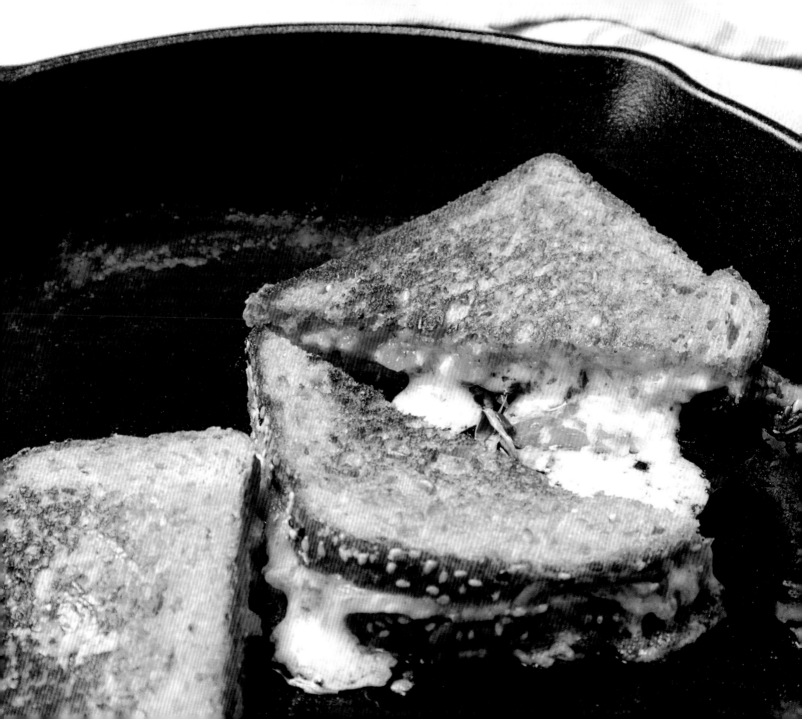

SALMON JERKY

Jerky has long been a go-to item when a snack attack strikes. A batch of habit-forming DIY salmon jerky is within reach without the hefty price tag of store-bought. All you need is a little planning and time. Then you'll be able to rip into a hunk of protein and omega-3-rich meat after any hard workout or pack it up and take it on the trail. The latest batch of studies suggests that mega-healthy omega-3 fats can help athletes boost immunity, reduce post-exercise muscle soreness, and perhaps even improve performance by bolstering blood flow.

SERVINGS: 8
ACTIVE TIME: 25 min.

Placing the salmon in the freezer for about 1 hour to firm it up before slicing makes it easier to slice the flesh thin. But don't let it freeze solid. Make this jerky even better by splurging for sustainable Pacific wild salmon.

1½ pounds skinless salmon, pin bones removed
1 cup orange juice
½ cup soy sauce, gluten-free if needed
2 tablespoons rice vinegar
2 garlic cloves, minced
2 tablespoons brown sugar or coconut sugar
1 tablespoon Asian chili sauce such as sriracha
1 tablespoon minced fresh ginger
1½ teaspoons liquid smoke (optional)
½ teaspoon cracked black pepper

Using a long, sharp chef's knife, slice fish into ¼-inch-thick strips (up to ½-inch max) that are 2 to 4 inches long. Mix together remaining ingredients in a large zip-top bag or shallow glass container. Add salmon, toss to coat, cover if using a glass container, and chill for 12 to 24 hours.

Turn oven to its lowest setting, no more than 225°F. Grease metal cooling racks and place them inside two large baking sheets. This allows air to flow on both sides of the meat, helping the jerky cook evenly. Drain off any excess marinade from salmon slices and arrange strips across the racks, leaving ¼ inch of space between each piece. (You can also place salmon directly on parchment paper–lined baking sheets, but be sure to flip the pieces once halfway through cooking.) Place sheets in the oven and wedge door open an inch with a dish towel or wooden spoon handle to allow moisture to escape, which helps the meat dry more evenly.

Start checking jerky after 2 hours. You want it to be dry but still chewy, not crunchy.

Rotate pans once halfway through cooking. Allow jerky to cool completely before storing in an airtight container in the refrigerator for up to 2 weeks.

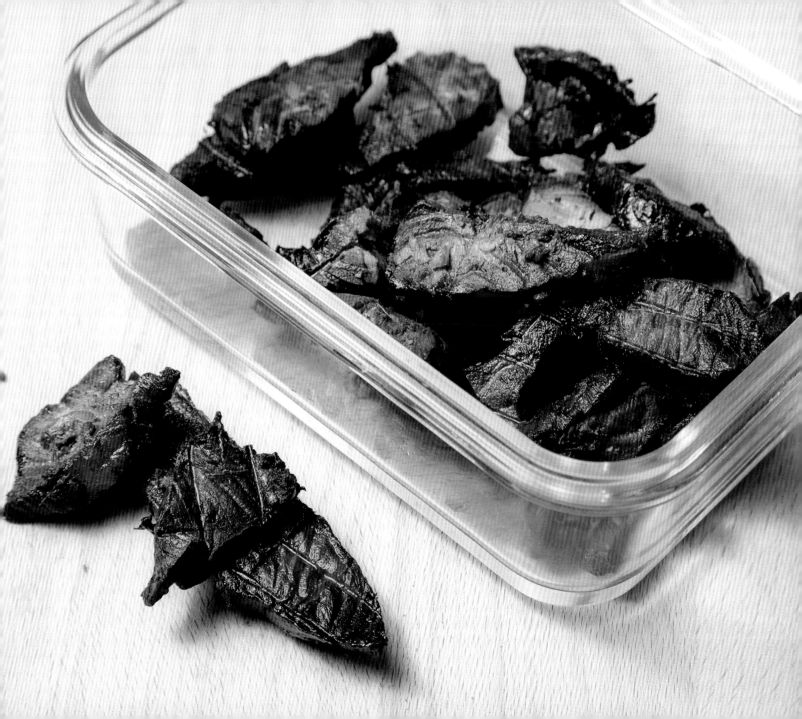

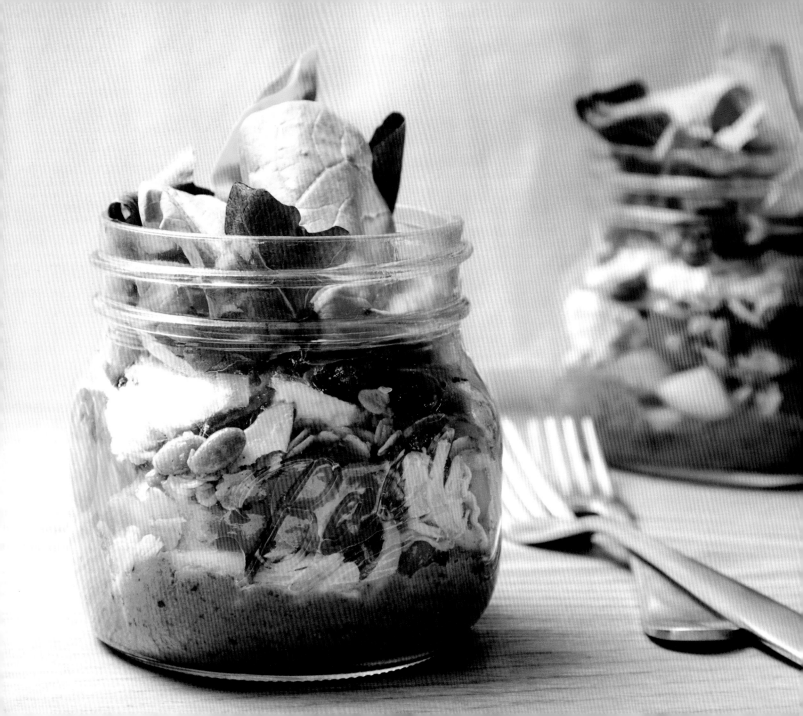

MUESLI SALAD

Most people should be eating more veggies, so why not work them and their nutrient payload into your post-training eating plan? With a tangy blueberry vinaigrette, ready-to-go roasted chicken, and crunchy muesli heated in a skillet until toasty, this ain't your run-of-the-mill rabbit food. It's also a standout lunch option for workdays.

D G

SERVINGS: 4
ACTIVE TIME: 25 min.

Packing this salad in jars lets you make portions ahead of time, allowing for quick nourishment following a workout or easy transport to the office. And by keeping the dressing down below the greens and muesli, you avoid any soggy ingredients. You can also apply the same stacking technique to bowls.

MUESLI

1 tablespoon coconut oil
1 tablespoon honey
¾ cup rolled oats
⅓ cup sliced almonds
¼ cup raw shelled pumpkin seeds (pepitas)
½ teaspoon cinnamon
¼ cup dried cherries

DRESSING

¾ cup fresh blueberries
3 tablespoons extra-virgin olive oil
2 tablespoons balsamic vinegar
2 teaspoons Dijon mustard
1 garlic clove, chopped

SALAD

8 ounces chopped rotisserie chicken (about 2 cups)
½ large English cucumber, chopped
1½ cups halved cherry tomatoes
3 ounces crumbled soft goat cheese (about 1 cup)
⅓ cup roughly chopped fresh mint
4 cups tender salad greens, such as baby spinach or mesclun

Heat coconut oil and honey in a skillet over medium heat until melted. Add rolled oats, almonds, pumpkin seeds, cinnamon, and a pinch of salt to the skillet and heat until oats are toasted, about 5 minutes, stirring frequently. Stir in cherries and spread mixture on a baking sheet or cutting board to cool.

Blend together blueberries, olive oil, 2 tablespoons water, balsamic vinegar, mustard, garlic, and salt and pepper to taste until smooth.

Divide dressing among 4 large wide-mouth glass jars. Add chicken, cucumber, tomatoes, muesli, goat cheese, mint, and salad greens, in that order. Seal shut and chill until ready to eat, or up to 4 days. To serve, turn the jar upside down and pour salad onto a serving plate, or if there is enough space in the jar, simply stir together the contents and dig in.

GAME CHANGERS Use oats labeled "gluten-free" or replace oats with quinoa flakes or spelt flakes + Swap out almonds for pecans or walnuts + Add protein with sliced pork tenderloin or cooked turkey breast instead of chicken + Use raspberries or blackberries for the dressing + Make it dairy-free by omitting goat cheese

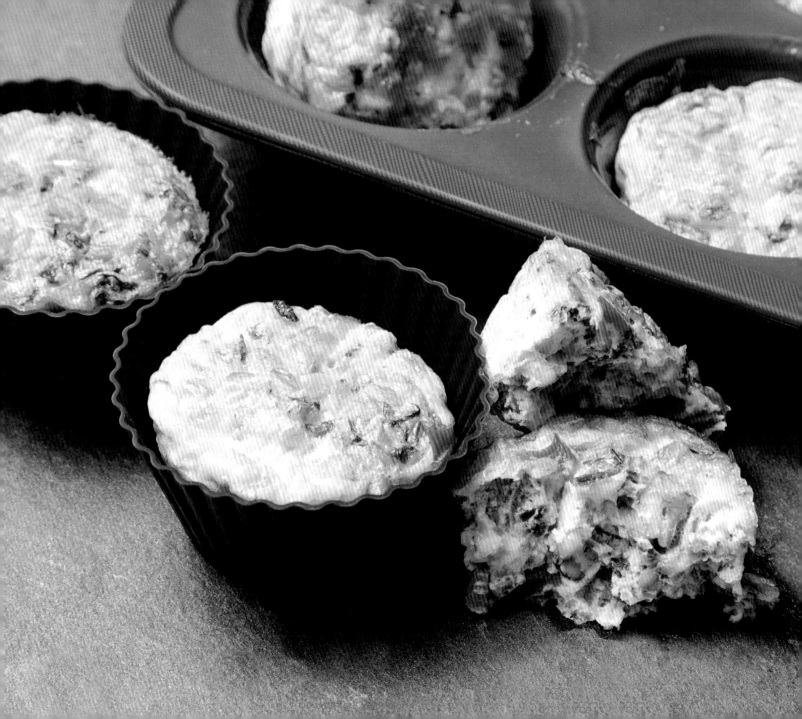

FARRO EGG CAKES

These egg cakes/handheld frittatas follow the rules of post-training nutrition, namely teaming up carbs and protein. You can enjoy them straight from the fridge or cooler, at room temperature, or heated for about 30 seconds in the microwave. And there is no reason why these can't serve as a quick breakfast or lunch option.

D G V

SERVINGS: 6
ACTIVE TIME: 20 min.

Baked eggs are tantamount to nature's version of cement, which is why I always break out my trusty silicone muffin tray so I don't have to chisel out the egg cakes once they're cooked.

Farro is a so-called ancient grain that can be found at an increasing number of natural food stores and megamarts.

½ cup farro
6 large eggs
⅓ cup low-fat milk
1 medium-sized red bell pepper, diced
1 cup finely chopped spinach
2 shallots, finely chopped
1 ounce grated Parmesan cheese (about ⅓ cup)
1 teaspoon dried thyme
1 teaspoon smoked paprika (optional)
½ teaspoon salt
¼ teaspoon black pepper

Place farro and 2 cups water in a medium-sized saucepan. Bring to a boil, reduce heat to medium-low, and simmer, covered, until grains are tender, about 25 minutes. Drain any excess water.

Preheat oven to 375°F. In a large bowl, whisk together eggs and milk. Stir in remaining ingredients and cooked farro. Divide among 12 standard-sized greased muffin cups and bake for 20 minutes, or until eggs are set. Let cool for a few minutes before unmolding. Keep chilled for up to 5 days.

GAME CHANGERS Swap out farro for wheat berries, freekeh, spelt, or for gluten-free, millet or sorghum + Make 'em dairy-free by using nondairy plain milk and replace Parmesan with nutritional yeast + Stir in chopped Swiss chard instead of spinach + Add some chopped cooked bacon

INSTANT MISO NOODLE SOUP

Full of salty liquid, this ready-to-go miso noodle soup is perfect for slurping up after working up a sweat—chopsticks optional! The best part is the flavorful broth you get to drink at the end. Turn it into an even bigger umami bomb by adding some dried seaweed or dried mushrooms. Brown rice vermicelli noodles are now available if you want a little extra nutrition in the jar.

SERVINGS: 1
ACTIVE TIME: 15 min.

Consider packing a few jars at once for several post-workout meals or to share with your workout mates.

2 teaspoons white or yellow miso paste
2 teaspoons reduced-sodium soy sauce
1 teaspoon sesame oil
1 teaspoon minced fresh ginger
½ teaspoon Chinese five-spice powder
½ teaspoon chili sauce, such as sriracha
1 ounce fine rice noodles (vermicelli), roughly chopped
1 hard-boiled egg, peeled and halved
1 small carrot, grated
½ cup baby spinach
1 scallion (green onion), thinly sliced
1 teaspoon sesame seeds

In a wide-mouth quart jar, whisk together miso paste, soy sauce, sesame oil, ginger, five-spice, and chili sauce. Top with noodles, egg, vegetables, and sesame seeds. Seal shut and refrigerate for up to 4 days until ready to use.

When ready to eat, fill the jar with boiling water, seal shut, and leave until the noodles are tender, 5 to 10 minutes.

GAME CHANGERS Replace soy sauce with gluten-free soy sauce, tamari, or liquid aminos + Add protein such as cooked chicken, cooked shrimp, or firm tofu instead of egg + Use chopped baby bok choy greens instead of spinach

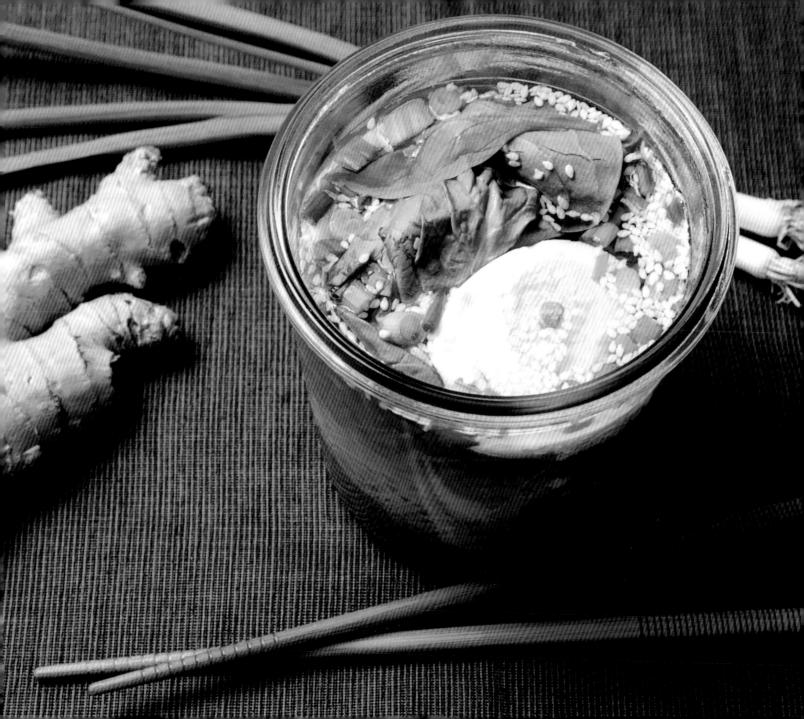

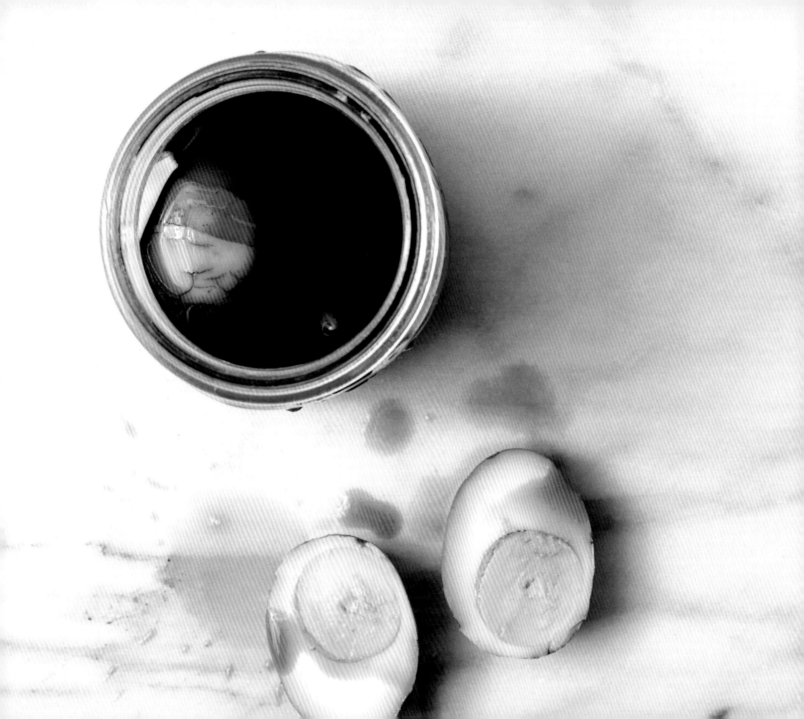

CHINESE PICKLED EGGS

If you've trained hard, you probably want your recovery protein to taste a little bit special. When protein-rich white orbs are imbued with a salty, vinegary snap, you've got a post-training item you'll race to the fridge for. Eggs are a rich source of leucine, an amino acid that is particularly effective at kick-starting muscle repair and building after workouts. If possible, opt for the more nutrient dense free-range eggs from a local supplier.

SERVINGS: 4
ACTIVE TIME: 15 min.

Don't pour the pickling liquid down the drain. It can be used to enliven another batch of eggs if it hasn't lingered in the fridge for weeks.

½ cup soy sauce
3 tablespoons rice vinegar
1 tablespoon honey
1 teaspoon Chinese five-spice powder
4 hard-boiled eggs, peeled
1 garlic clove, smashed

Place soy sauce, rice vinegar, honey, and five-spice powder in a small saucepan. Heat over medium heat, stirring until honey has dissolved. Remove from heat and let cool.

Place hard-boiled eggs and garlic in a large jar, pour soy sauce mixture over top, and add enough water to just cover the eggs. Seal top, place jar in the refrigerator, and let chill for several hours (and up to 1 week total) before consuming.

GAME CHANGERS Use liquid aminos or gluten-free soy sauce instead of regular soy sauce + Replace five-spice powder with a whole star anise

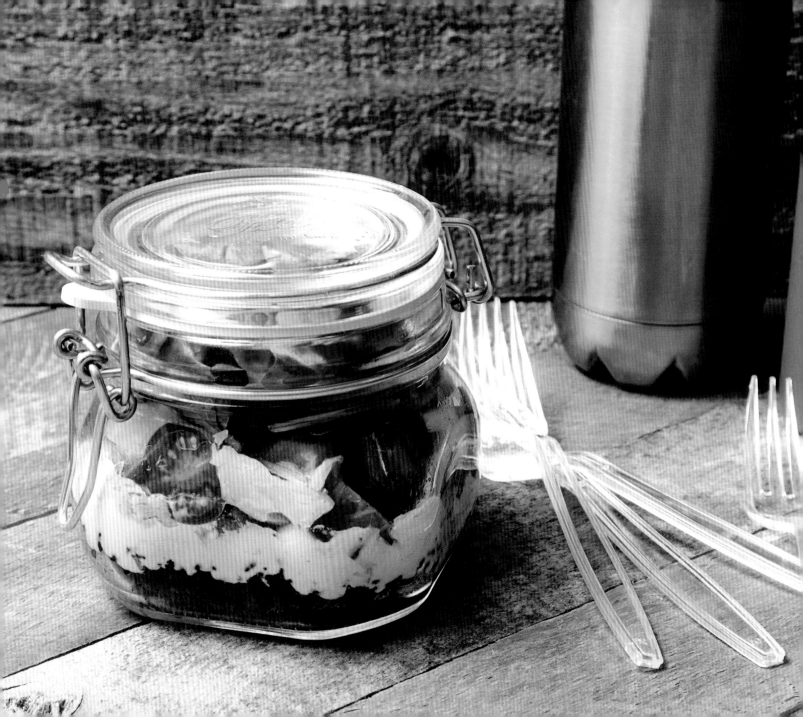

SALMON SALAD JARS

If I know I'll be pushing my pedals all day and am bound to return home late with little energy to rustle up a meal, I'll break out my jars the day before and stuff them full of this mélange of nutritional bell-ringers. Protein, healthy carbs, omega fats—it's a recovery-worthy repast indeed. I often double the recipe (4 jars) so my girlfriend and I are taken care of for a couple of meals, giving us more time to enjoy the open road.

G

SERVINGS: 2
ACTIVE TIME: 20 min.

Also sold under the trademarked name Forbidden Rice, black rice is an heirloom variety of rice from China that has a wonderful chew and subtle sweetness as well as higher antioxidant values than brown rice. Look for it in health food shops, Asian grocers, or at www.lotusfoods.com.

½ cup black rice (Forbidden Rice)
½ avocado
½ cup plain yogurt
  Juice of ½ lime
1 garlic clove, chopped
1 teaspoon Asian hot sauce, such as sriracha
1 cup halved cherry tomatoes
1 cup diced pineapple
½ English cucumber, chopped
1 scallion (green onion), thinly sliced
¼ cup roughly chopped fresh mint
½ pound cooked salmon, flesh broken apart
2 cups baby spinach

Place rice and 1 cup water in a small saucepan. Bring to a boil, reduce heat, and simmer, covered, until rice is tender, about 20 minutes. Remove from heat and let stand, covered, for 5 minutes. Fluff with a fork.

Blend together avocado, yogurt, lime juice, garlic, hot sauce, and a pinch of salt until smooth. In a bowl, toss together tomatoes, pineapple, cucumber, scallion, mint, and a pinch of salt.

Divide cooked rice among 2 large wide-mouth glass jars. Add avocado sauce, cooked salmon, tomato mixture, and spinach, in that order. Seal shut and chill until ready to eat, for up to 2 days. To serve, turn the jar upside down and pour salad onto a serving plate or, if there is enough space in the jar, simply stir together the contents and dig in.

GAME CHANGERS   Swap out black rice for brown rice or quinoa ✦ Replace yogurt with reduced-fat sour cream ✦ Use rainbow trout, arctic char, smoked salmon, or a good-quality canned salmon instead of fresh salmon ✦ Top with arugula or baby kale in lieu of spinach

POTATO PANCAKE SMOKED FISH SANDWICHES

Incorporating some salmon into your post-workout routine not only provides protein but also gives you a shot of omega-3 fatty acids, which have been linked to reduced muscle soreness and even reduced body fat levels in response to exercise. Stir a tablespoon of prepared horseradish into the lemony cream cheese for a little kick. You could also simply slather some apple butter or walnut butter onto the potato pancakes as an exercise nosh option.

D G

SERVINGS: 8
ACTIVE TIME: 25 min.

For a taste of sustainability, seek out smoked salmon sourced from a healthy wild salmon population, such as those swimming in Alaskan waters.

1 pound russet or Yukon Gold potatoes, peeled and cubed
2 large eggs, lightly beaten
½ cup all-purpose flour
¼ cup low-fat milk
2 tablespoons chopped fresh chives
1 teaspoon garlic powder
½ teaspoon baking powder
½ teaspoon salt
1 tablespoon grapeseed, canola, or light olive oil
4 ounces cream cheese (about ½ cup)
2 teaspoons lemon zest
4 ounces smoked salmon

Steam or boil potatoes until very tender. Drain if boiling, place in a large bowl, and mash until smooth. Let cool and then stir in eggs, flour, milk, chives, garlic powder, baking powder, and salt. The mixture will be fairly sticky.

Heat oil in a skillet over medium heat. For each pancake, scoop about 1½ tablespoons of potato batter into the pan and flatten into a pancake using a spatula or the back of a spoon. Don't worry if they are not perfectly round. Heat 2 minutes per side, or until golden on both sides. Remove pancakes from pan and let cool on wire racks. Repeat with remaining batter, adding more oil as needed. You will end up with 16 to 18 pancakes. The unassembled pancakes will keep in the fridge for about 5 days.

Stir together cream cheese and lemon zest. To assemble, spread about 1 tablespoon cream cheese on a pancake. Top with some smoked fish and another pancake. The pancakes are best assembled no more than a day in advance of consuming.

GAME CHANGERS Swap out the white spuds for sweet potatoes + Use gluten-free flour instead of all-purpose flour + Spread on dairy-free cream cheese, goat cheese, or pesto instead of cream cheese + Stuff with smoked trout or smoked mackerel instead of salmon

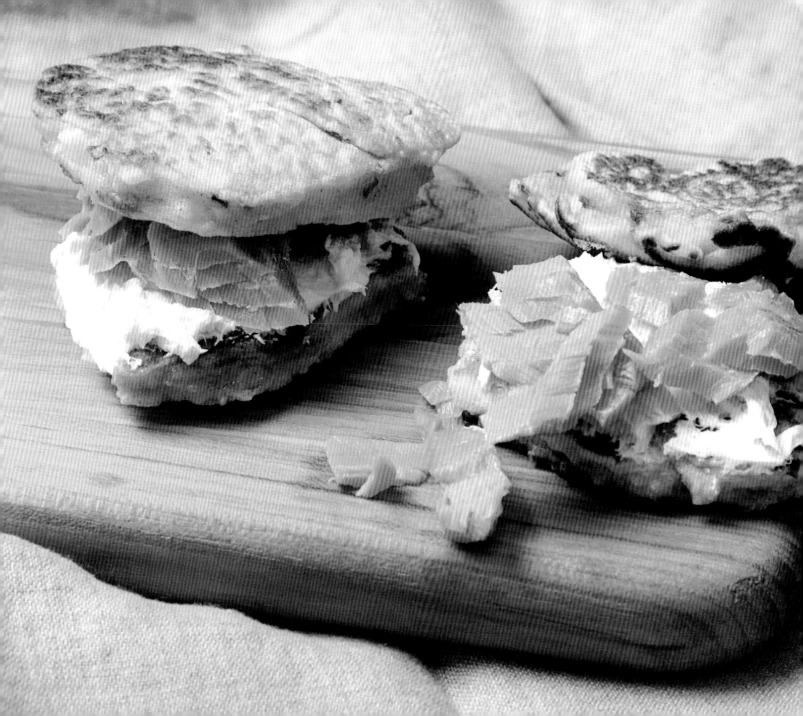

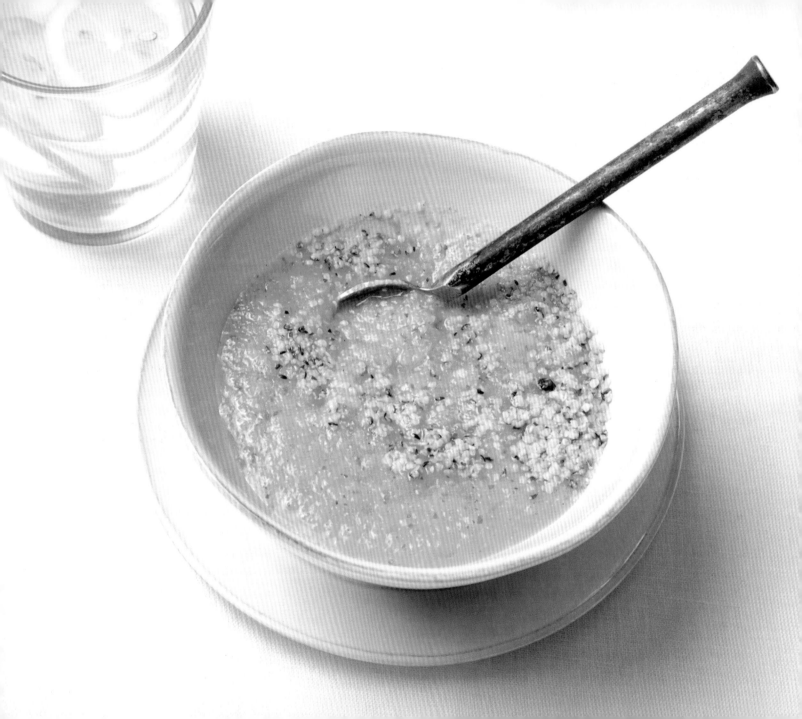

APRICOT GAZPACHO

Gazpacho is an iconic cold soup featuring tomatoes. This riff uses apricots for a wonderful sweet-savory combo, and it provides a powerful mix of carbohydrates, vitamins, minerals, antioxidants, and fluid to support exercise recovery. Antioxidants delivered in natural amounts via fruits and vegetables (not the mega doses from supplements) have been thought to lessen the muscle cell–damaging impact of intense exercise, thereby playing a big part in the recovery process. Sprinkle on some nutty-tasting hemp seeds for a hit of protein. Other garnish options include diced avocado or even fresh lump crabmeat. You can also blend in a couple of yellow or orange tomatoes, especially when local heirloom varieties are in season.

SERVINGS: 4
ACTIVE TIME: 15 min.

To spoon up this gazpacho immediately after a workout or race, place a portion in a jar and transport in a cooler. Give the jar a shake before serving, as separation may occur.

⅔ cup water
1 pound fresh apricots (about 6 to 8), pitted and quartered
1 medium-sized orange bell pepper, roughly chopped
½ English cucumber, chopped
2 scallions (green onions), white and green parts, sliced
1 garlic clove, chopped
2 teaspoons chopped fresh ginger
3 tablespoons fresh mint
2 tablespoons red wine vinegar or white wine vinegar
¼ teaspoon sea salt
¼ teaspoon black pepper
2 tablespoons extra-virgin olive oil or almond oil
8 tablespoons hemp seeds

Place all of the ingredients except for the oil and hemp seeds in a blender or food processor and blend until smooth. With the machine running on low speed, pour in oil through the top feed tube until it's incorporated into the soup. Chill in the refrigerator for at least 2 hours before serving. Serve each bowlful topped with 2 tablespoons hemp seeds. Can be kept chilled for up to 5 days.

GAME CHANGERS Use peaches instead of apricots ✦ Swap out mint for fresh basil ✦ Top with chopped pistachios instead of hemp seeds

TURKEY MUFFINS

If your workout was dominated by a sweet deluge of gels and chews, these savory muffins will offer your palate a shred of comfort. They're a tasty reward for getting through a tough workout, and they also contain a notable amount of protein to fire up muscle recovery and growth. They're especially good when warmed in the microwave and then adorned with a touch of butter.

F G

SERVINGS: 12
ACTIVE TIME: 20 min.

These muffins contain meat, so make sure to store them in the fridge or a cooler if transporting them. Lower-fat lean ground turkey is sometimes labeled "ground turkey breast."

2 teaspoons + ¼ cup canola, grapeseed, or light olive oil
1 pound lean ground turkey
1½ cups whole wheat pastry flour
1 tablespoon dried sage or 2 tablespoons chopped fresh sage
2 teaspoons garlic powder
1 tablespoon sugar
1 teaspoon baking powder
¼ teaspoon baking soda
2 large eggs
1 cup grated Parmesan cheese
1¼ cups 2% plain yogurt

Heat 2 teaspoons oil in a skillet over medium heat. Add turkey and cook until no longer pink, breaking up the meat into small pieces as it cooks. Remove turkey from pan and let cool.

Preheat oven to 350°F. In a large bowl, mix together flour, sage, garlic powder, sugar, baking powder, and baking soda. In a separate bowl, lightly beat eggs. Stir in cheese, yogurt, and ¼ cup oil. Add wet ingredients to dry ingredients and mix gently. Fold in cooked turkey.

Divide mixture among 12 standard-sized silicone or greased metal muffin cups and bake for 20 minutes, or until a toothpick inserted into the center of a muffin comes out nearly clean. Let cool for a few minutes before unmolding and cooling completely on metal racks. Chill for up to 5 days or freeze for up to 1 month.

GAME CHANGERS Replace ground turkey with cooked turkey sausage or ground chicken + Use spelt flour, all-purpose flour, or 1-to-1 gluten-free flour blend instead of whole wheat pastry flour + Switch out sage for thyme or chopped fresh rosemary + Use sour cream in lieu of yogurt

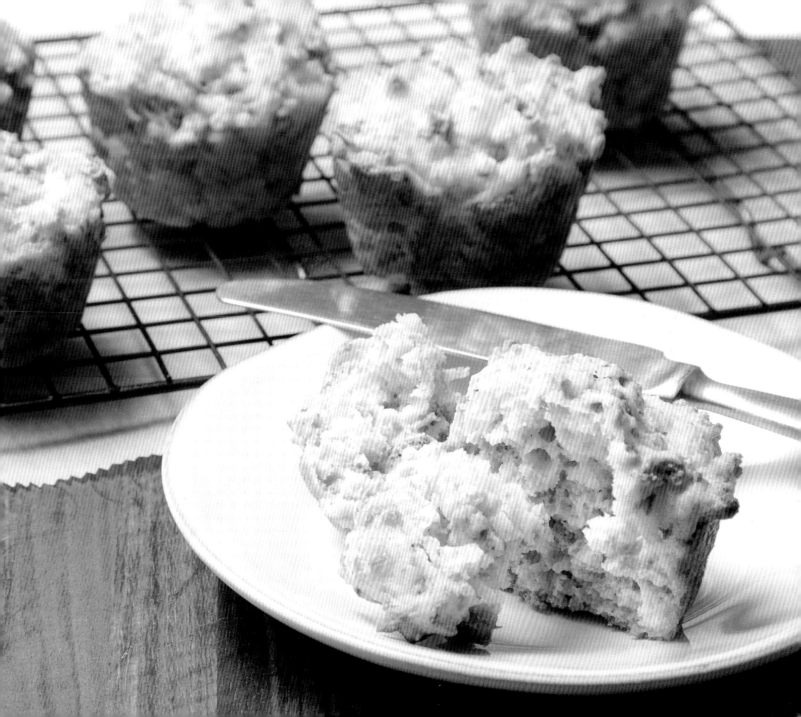

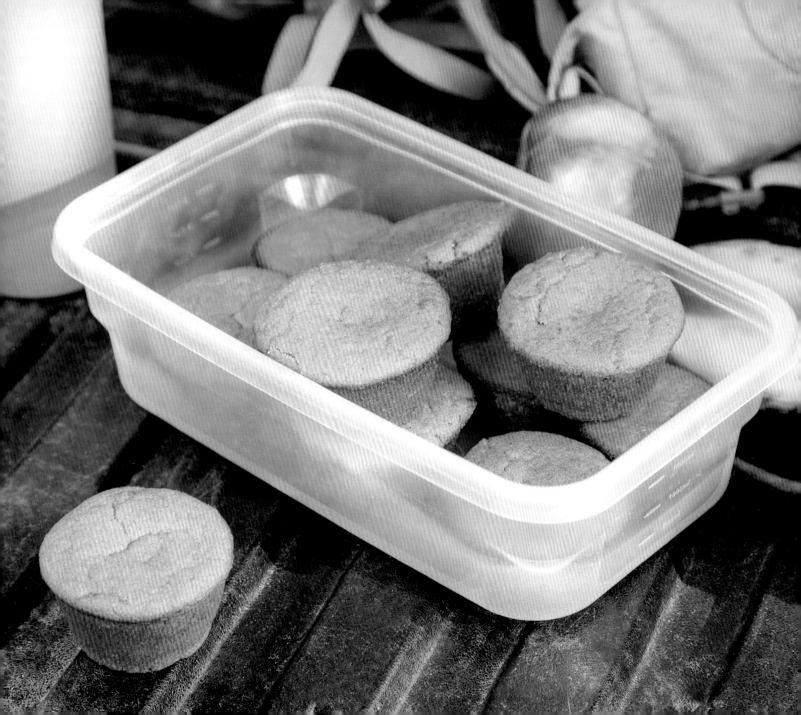

FLOURLESS PROTEIN BANANA MUFFINS

These portable, protein-rich muffins remove the "woulda coulda shoulda" from kick-starting recovery quickly after a lively workout. Dried cherries add a shot of muscle-mending antioxidants.

D F G P V

SERVINGS: 12
ACTIVE TIME: 20 min.

The best bananas for this recipe are ones with a considerable amount of black on the skin. You can expedite ripening by baking the bananas with the skin still intact in a 250ºF oven for 15 to 20 minutes.

Using too much whey protein, more than about 30 percent of the total amount of flour in a recipe, can result in overly rubbery muffins. For this reason, I prefer using a plant-based protein powder such as rice or hemp in baked goods.

- 3 large eggs
- ⅓ cup low-fat milk
- 3 medium-sized ripe bananas
- ¼ cup honey
- 1¾ cups almond flour
- ½ cup plain or vanilla protein powder
- 1 teaspoon cinnamon
- ¾ teaspoon ground ginger
- ½ teaspoon baking soda
- ½ teaspoon baking powder
- ¼ teaspoon salt
- ½ cup roughly chopped dried cherries

Preheat oven to 350ºF. Place all of the ingredients except for the dried cherries in a blender or food processor and blend until smooth. Scrape down sides as needed during blending. Stir in cherries.

Divide batter among 12 standard-sized greased or paper-lined muffin cups. Bake until set and lightly browned on top and a toothpick inserted into the center of a muffin comes out nearly clean, about 22 to 25 minutes. Let cool for a few minutes before unmolding and cooling completely on metal racks. Chill for up to 5 days.

GAME CHANGERS Instead of cow milk, use plain nondairy milk such as almond or hemp ✦ Use maple syrup in lieu of honey ✦ Swap out almond flour for hazelnut flour ✦ Stir in chocolate chips instead of cherries

SPAGHETTI BOLOGNESE MUFFINS

Here's a fun way to enjoy an athlete's favorite pasta with meat sauce—and the recovery-accelerating carb-protein duo it provides—almost instantly after your cooldown. If there is more pasta mixture than you can fit into your muffin cups, you can prepare the muffins in two batches.

D F G

SERVINGS: 12
ACTIVE TIME: 30 min.

You can enjoy these straight from the fridge or cooler, or warm them up in the microwave or toaster oven. To freeze for later use, place the pasta cups on a baking sheet and freeze until solid. Transfer frozen spaghetti muffins to an airtight container and stash in the freezer for up to 1 month.

½ pound spaghetti, broken in half
1 pound lean ground beef
4 large eggs, lightly beaten
2 cups tomato sauce
1 cup grated Parmesan cheese
2 teaspoons dried oregano
1 teaspoon onion powder
1 teaspoon garlic powder
½ teaspoon salt
½ teaspoon red chili flakes (optional)

Bring a large pot of water to a boil. Add pasta and cook until al dente, about 7 minutes. Drain well.

Preheat oven to 350°F and grease 12 standard-sized muffin cups. Cook beef in a skillet until no longer pink, breaking up the meat as it cooks. Stir in cooked spaghetti, eggs, tomato sauce, Parmesan, oregano, onion powder, garlic powder, salt, and chili flakes, if using.

Divide pasta mixture among muffin cups and tightly pack in contents to help everything hold together. Bake for 20 minutes and then let cool for several minutes before unmolding. Let cool completely on metal racks before storing in an airtight container in the refrigerator for up to 4 days.

GAME CHANGERS Replace regular spaghetti with gluten-free noodles ◆ Use ground turkey, chicken, or even bison instead of beef ◆ Season with dried basil instead of oregano ◆ For dairy-free, omit the Parmesan cheese

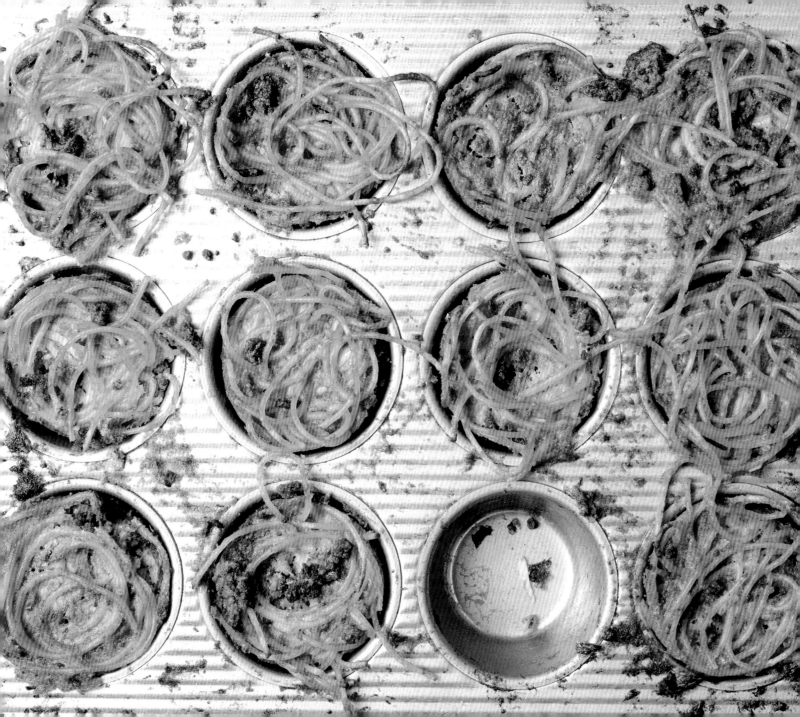

PIZZA MUG CAKE

Why tip the delivery guy when you can use a coffee mug and microwave to turn your post-training period into a pizza party, minus the need to crank up the oven? The marriage of carbs, protein, and sodium makes this pizza mug cake a delicious way to send forth recovery.

G V

SERVINGS: 1
ACTIVE TIME: 10 min.

Not a coffee drinker? You can also nuke the pizza cake in ramekins, a small microwave-safe cereal bowl, or silicone muffin cups—no metal, please!

¼ cup all-purpose flour
½ teaspoon garlic powder
½ teaspoon onion powder
¼ teaspoon baking powder
⅛ teaspoon baking soda
1 tablespoon chopped fresh basil
¼ cup low-fat milk
1 tablespoon olive oil
2 teaspoons tomato paste
2 tablespoons chopped pepperette or pepperoni
3 tablespoons shredded mozzarella cheese, divided

Grease the inside of a medium or large coffee mug with oil or cooking spray. Place flour, garlic powder, onion powder, baking powder, and baking soda in bowl and stir to combine. Stir in basil, milk, olive oil, tomato paste, pepperette or pepperoni, and 2 tablespoons cheese. Pour into the mug and top with remaining 1 tablespoon cheese.

Cover mug with paper towel and microwave on high until puffed and set, about 90 seconds to 2 minutes, depending on the power of your machine.

Serve straight from the mug or use a butter knife to loosen the edges of the cake and dump onto a plate.

GAME CHANGERS Swap out all-purpose flour for whole wheat pastry flour, spelt flour, or 1-to-1 gluten-free flour blend ✦ Use ½ teaspoon dried Italian seasoning instead of fresh basil ✦ Blend in shredded cheddar cheese in place of mozzarella

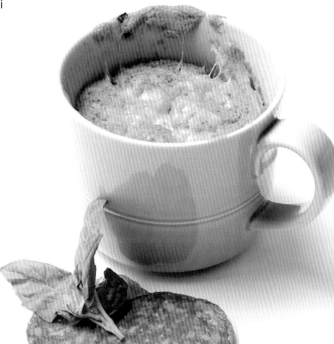

MOLTEN CHOCOLATE MUG CAKE

This ready-in-a-hurry moist cake lets you throw down the calories, carbs, and protein your muscles need after a workout. Of course, it also makes for a quick dessert fix for chocoholics. For a splash of color, you can top the cake with raspberries or sliced strawberries.

SERVINGS: 1
ACTIVE TIME: 10 min.

As with most cakes, muffins, and other baked goods, consider using a plant-based protein such as rice or hemp. It produces a better texture than whey.

1 egg
3 tablespoons plain yogurt
2 teaspoons almond butter or other nut butter
1 tablespoon brown sugar
½ teaspoon instant espresso powder (optional)
2 tablespoons all-purpose flour
2 tablespoons protein powder
1 tablespoon cocoa powder
1 tablespoon dried tart cherries (optional)
¼ teaspoon cinnamon
¼ teaspoon baking soda

Grease the inside of a coffee mug with oil or cooking spray. Stir together egg, yogurt, nut butter, sugar, and espresso powder (if using), in a bowl. Stir in flour, protein powder, cocoa powder, dried tart cherries (if using), cinnamon, baking soda, and a pinch of salt. Mix well until smooth and then pour into the mug.

Cover mug with a paper towel and microwave on high until puffed and set, about 90 seconds to 2 minutes, depending on the power of your machine. Eat straight from mug or use a butter knife to loosen and turn out onto a plate.

GAME CHANGERS Swap out regular yogurt for a dairy-free yogurt + Replace brown sugar with coconut sugar or turbinado sugar + Use whole wheat pastry flour, spelt flour, or 1-to-1 gluten-free flour blend instead of all-purpose flour

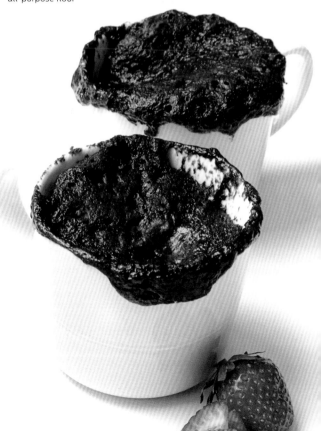

CHERRY MOJITO POPSICLES

A raft of research trumpets the antioxidants in tart cherries for improving exercise recovery, mainly by limiting inflammation and muscle damage in the body. These cocktail-inspired popsicles are a refreshing way to work both recovery-boosting tart cherry juice and protein-laced Greek yogurt into your post-workout routine. They are also a great treat for kids after a sports practice. On the flip side, if you want to make these slightly boozy, mix a couple tablespoons of rum into the cherry mixture.

SERVINGS: 6
ACTIVE TIME: 15 min.

You can also use tart cherry concentrate for this recipe. Simply combine 3 tablespoons of the syrupy concentrate with 1¼ cups water.

1¼ cups plain Greek yogurt
2 tablespoons honey
Zest of 1 lime
1¼ cups tart cherry juice
Juice of 1 lime
⅓ cup finely chopped fresh mint leaves

Stir together yogurt, honey, and lime zest. In a separate bowl, stir together cherry juice, lime juice, and mint.

Spoon two alternate layers of yogurt and cherry mixture into each popsicle mold. Insert popsicle sticks into the molds and freeze until solid, about 6 hours.

To unmold the popsicles, run the mold under warm water for a few seconds, being careful not to thaw the pops. Store in the freezer for up to 2 months.

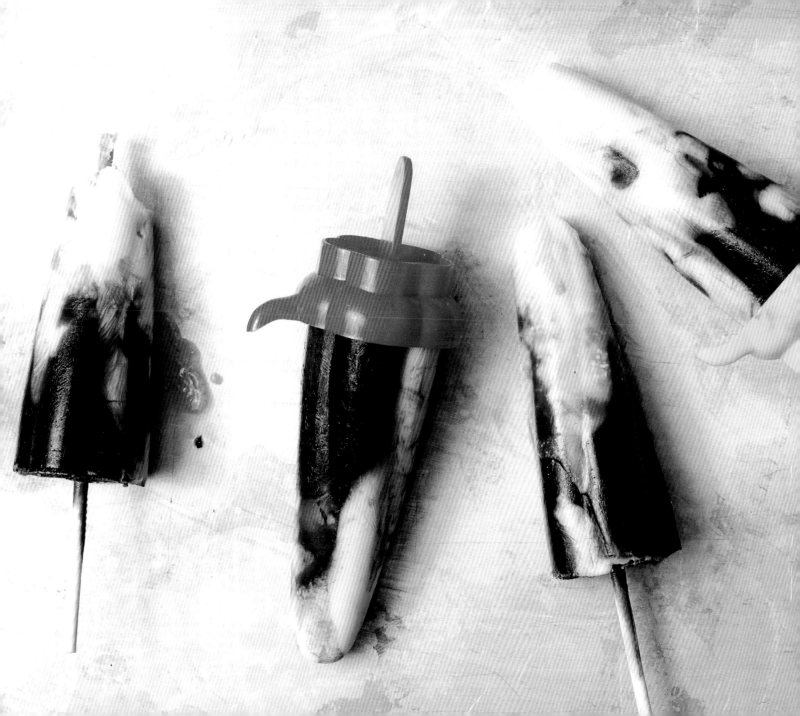

RECOVERY ICE CREAM

Frozen banana sent for a whirl in the food processor (or a high-powered blender) produces deliciously silky ice cream–like results. No ice cream maker required! It's a great way to cool down and reboot after a sticky workout. For added carbs and crunch, sprinkle on some granola.

SERVINGS: 1
ACTIVE TIME: 5 min.

To freeze bananas for ice cream or smoothies, peel and chop the ripe fruit into 1-inch chunks. Spread out on a baking sheet and place in the freezer until solid, 2 or more hours.

Stick your serving bowl in the freezer before heading out for a workout to delay the time it takes the ice cream to melt after serving.

1 large or 2 small frozen bananas, cut into chunks

PB&J

1 tablespoon peanut butter
4–6 strawberries or ½ cup raspberries
¼ cup plain or vanilla protein powder
½ teaspoon vanilla extract (omit if using vanilla protein)

MINT CHIP

½ cup plain low-fat Greek yogurt or nondairy yogurt
2 tablespoons mini–chocolate chips
1 tablespoon coconut butter (optional)
¼ teaspoon peppermint extract

PEACH CHEESECAKE

1 peach, quartered
½ cup reduced-fat ricotta cheese
1 tablespoon almond butter
1 teaspoon lemon zest (optional)
¼ teaspoon cinnamon

GOTCHA MATCHA

1 teaspoon matcha tea powder
¼ cup plain or vanilla protein powder
2 teaspoons honey
¼ teaspoon ground ginger

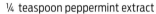

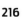

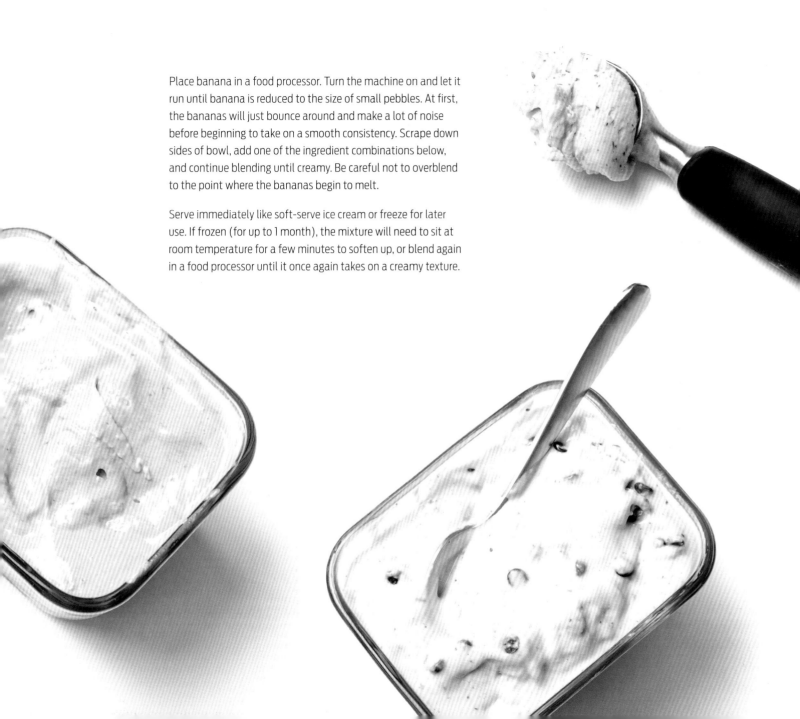

Place banana in a food processor. Turn the machine on and let it run until banana is reduced to the size of small pebbles. At first, the bananas will just bounce around and make a lot of noise before beginning to take on a smooth consistency. Scrape down sides of bowl, add one of the ingredient combinations below, and continue blending until creamy. Be careful not to overblend to the point where the bananas begin to melt.

Serve immediately like soft-serve ice cream or freeze for later use. If frozen (for up to 1 month), the mixture will need to sit at room temperature for a few minutes to soften up, or blend again in a food processor until it once again takes on a creamy texture.

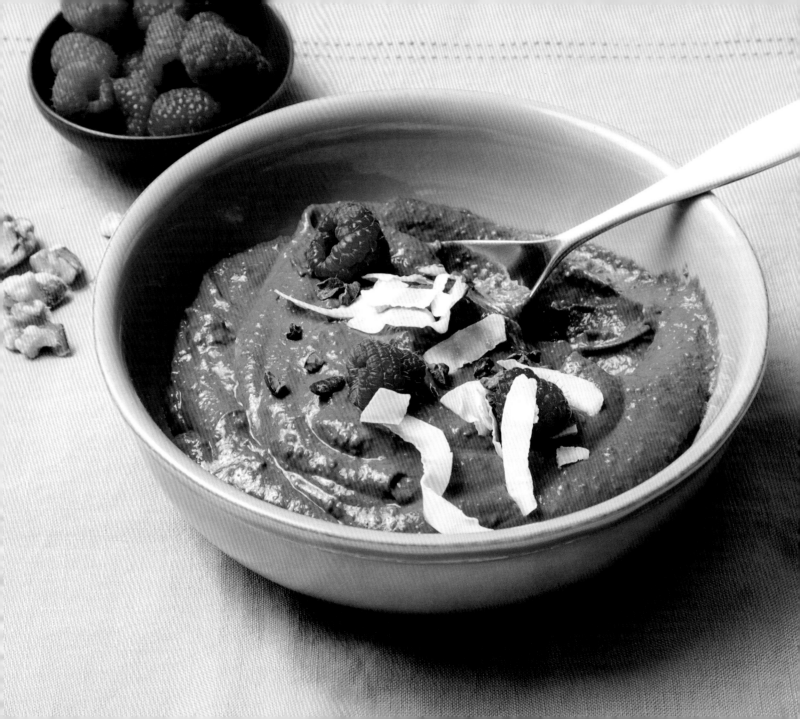

CHOCOLATE AVOCADO PUDDING

Just the thought of rewarding yourself with this creamy and chocolaty delight will help motivate you to push harder. Each spoonful provides a great mix of carbs, protein, and healthy fats. And tasters would never be the wiser of its nutrient-dense avocado origins. Garnish options run the gamut, from dried coconut, walnuts, raspberries, sliced mango, cacao nibs, or granola.

`D G P V`

SERVINGS: 4
ACTIVE TIME: 15 min.

A nearly foolproof way to tell whether your avocado is pudding-ready is to peel back the small stem at the top. If you see green underneath, the avocado is likely at its creamy best. Brown under the stem is a sign the fruit is overripe and likely past its prime. If the stem resists removing, the avocado is not yet ripe enough for use.

⅓ cup low-fat milk

2 avocados, pitted and flesh scooped out

2 medium-sized bananas

½ cup plain or vanilla protein powder

⅓ cup unsweetened cocoa powder

¼ cup pure maple syrup

1 teaspoon vanilla extract (omit if using vanilla protein powder)

1 teaspoon instant espresso powder (optional)

½ teaspoon cinnamon

⅛ teaspoon salt

Place all of the ingredients in a blender or food processor and blend until smooth. If needed, add a small amount of additional milk to help with blending. Divide between 4 bowls if serving immediately or jars if storing. Keeps for up to 3 days in the refrigerator.

GAME CHANGERS Instead of cow milk, use a plain nondairy alternative ✦ Try brewed and cooled coffee instead of milk ✦ Add ½ cup melted dark chocolate chips in place of cocoa powder ✦ Swap out maple syrup for honey, brown rice syrup, or agave syrup

GRANOLA PIE

What happens when you morph granola into pie? Boom ... a post-workout nosh that steals the show. This is a great make-ahead dish that can feed a hungry crowd after a group run or ride. It's also a stellar breakfast option when you need to get out the door fast. As with most granola recipes, this pie version is highly customizable based on what nuts and dried fruit are in your pantry. Heck, why not forgo the yogurt and top with a few dollops of Recovery Ice Cream (p. 216)?

D F G V

SERVINGS: 8
ACTIVE TIME: 20 min.

Wedges of pie are best served warmed, which is as easy as zapping them in the microwave for about 35 seconds.

1½ cups rolled oats
⅓ cup buckwheat flour
⅓ cup chopped walnuts
⅓ cup chopped hazelnuts
⅓ cup chopped dried apricots
⅓ cup dried currants
3 tablespoons hemp seeds (optional)
1 teaspoon baking powder
1 teaspoon cinnamon
1 teaspoon ground ginger (optional)
¼ teaspoon salt
2 large eggs
½ cup unsweetened applesauce
⅓ cup pure maple syrup
¼ cup melted coconut oil
2 cups plain or vanilla Greek yogurt

Preheat oven to 325°F. Line the bottom of an 8- or 9-inch round cake pan with parchment paper and lightly grease the sides.

In a large bowl, stir together oats, buckwheat flour, nuts, dried fruit, hemp seeds (if using), baking powder, cinnamon, ginger (if using), and salt.
In a separate bowl, lightly beat the eggs and stir in applesauce, maple syrup, and oil. Add wet ingredients to dry mixture and mix until everything is moist.

Place mixture in pan and press down into an even layer. Bake for 30 minutes, or until edges are golden and center is set. Let cool in pan for several minutes before slicing into wedges. Serve topped with dollops of yogurt. Granola pie can be made and chilled up to 5 days in advance.

GAME CHANGERS Use oats labeled "gluten-free" or replace oats with quinoa flakes or spelt flakes ✦ Swap out buckwheat flour for oat flour ✦ Use almonds or pecans instead of hazelnuts or walnuts ✦ Stir in dried cherries or raisins instead of currants ✦ Sweeten with honey in lieu of maple syrup ✦ Replace coconut oil with a neutral-tasting oil such as canola or grapeseed ✦ Top with dollops of dairy-free yogurt instead of Greek

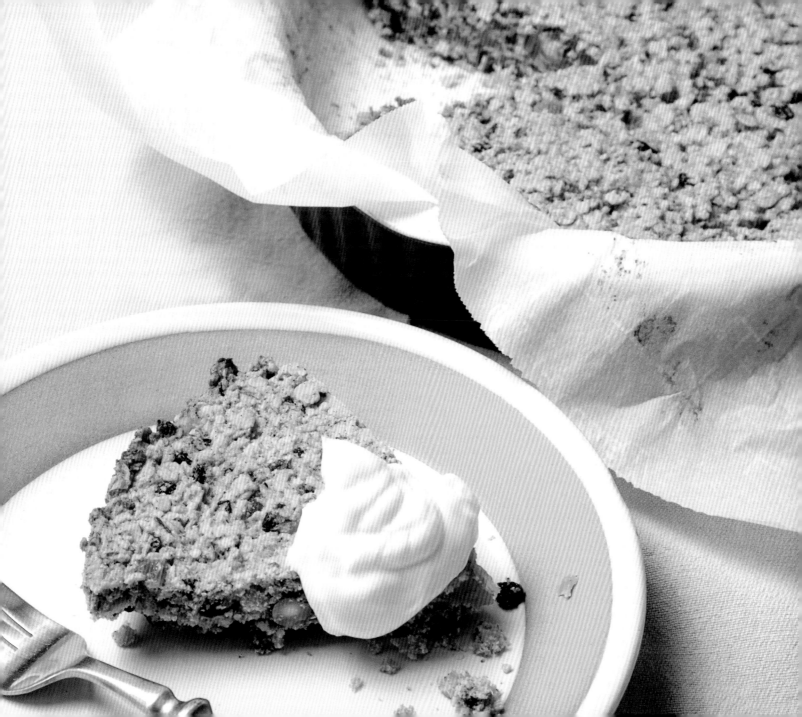

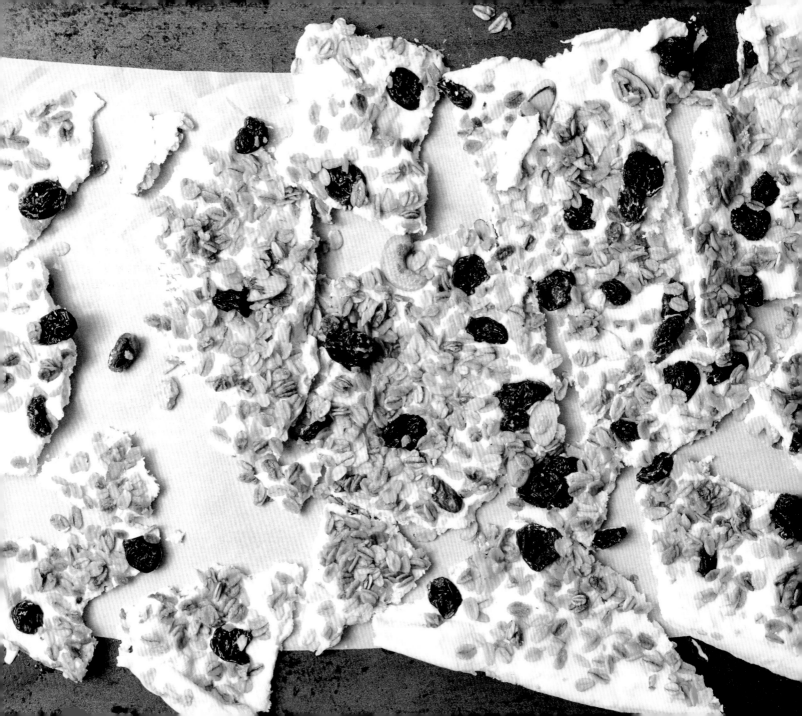

GRANOLA YOGURT BARK

In the throes of summer, all generations of a household will enjoy cooling down with this yogurt bark, which provides a winning mix of protein, carbs, and anti-inflammatory antioxidants (*merci*, tart cherries). If you've just finished up a run on asphalt that was seemingly on fire, you'll appreciate having these frosty chunks ready to welcome you home.

SERVINGS: 6
ACTIVE TIME: 10 min.

I prefer not to use fat-free yogurt for this recipe since a little bit of fat gives the frozen bark a creamier mouthfeel and reduces the formation of ice crystals.

- 2 cups plain 2% Greek yogurt
- 2 tablespoons honey
- 2 teaspoons vanilla extract
- 2 teaspoons orange zest (optional)
- ⅓ cup dried tart cherries
- 1 cup granola

Stir together yogurt, honey, vanilla, orange zest (if using), and a pinch of salt. Line a baking sheet with parchment paper or a silicone baking mat. Spread out yogurt mixture about ½-inch thick. Sprinkle on tart cherries and granola and press down gently to help them adhere.

Place sheet in freezer until set, about 1 hour. Break bark into desired-sized pieces and store in an airtight container or bag in the freezer for up to 1 month.

GAME CHANGERS Use vanilla yogurt and omit honey and vanilla extract ✦ Replace dried cherries with dried cranberries or fresh blueberries ✦ Swap out granola for chopped nuts

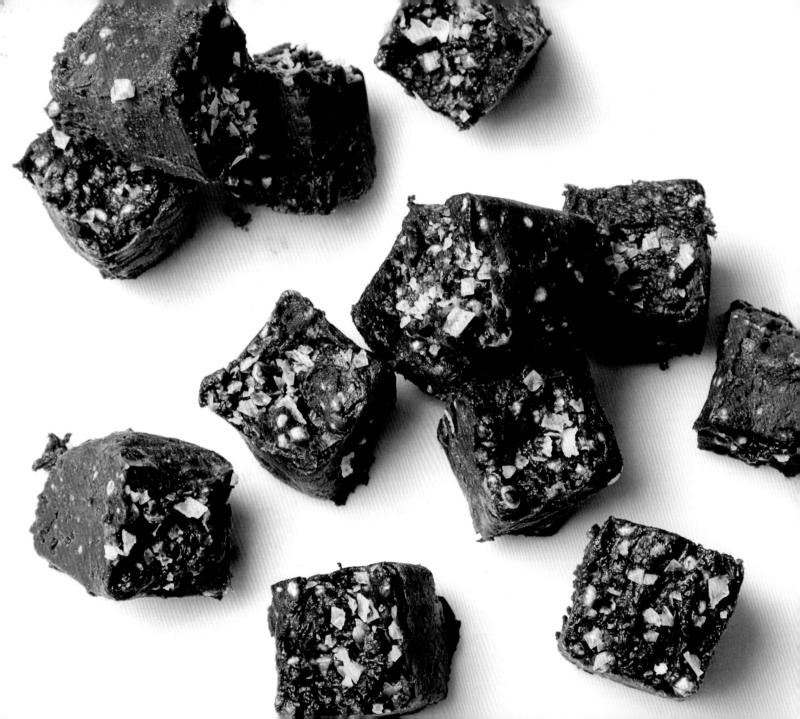

SALTED QUINOA ALMOND FUDGE CUPS

Every good deed deserves a reward. So after a health-boosting workout, why not luxuriate in some fudge? Of course, this version has more of what you need to recover well than any typical store-bought fudge. Case in point: I've worked in some protein powder, banana, and quinoa puffs for extra recovery protein and carbohydrates.

SERVINGS: 12

ACTIVE TIME: 20 min.

No mini-muffin tray? You can also mold the fudge in lightly greased ice cube trays. You may need to use a butter knife to unmold the set fudge pieces.

½ cup almond butter
½ cup protein powder
⅓ cup softened coconut oil
¼ cup cocoa powder
¼ cup pure maple syrup
1 medium-sized ripe banana
1 teaspoon vanilla extract
1 teaspoon cinnamon
1 cup quinoa puffs
1 teaspoon flaky salt, such as fleur de sel or Maldon

Place almond butter, protein powder, coconut oil, cocoa powder, maple syrup, banana, vanilla, and cinnamon in a food processor or blender and blend until smooth. Pulse in quinoa puffs.

Divide mixture among 24 silicone mini-muffin cups or paper-lined metal mini-muffin cups. Sprinkle salt over tops. Place tray in freezer until set, about 1 hour. The fudge cups will remain fairly soft and won't freeze solid. Unmold fudge cups and keep in an airtight container or zip-top bag in the freezer for up to 1 month. They can also be transported to an event in a cooler.

GAME CHANGERS Swap out almond butter for peanut butter + Sweeten with brown rice syrup or honey instead of maple syrup + Replace quinoa puffs with other small cereal puffs, such as millet

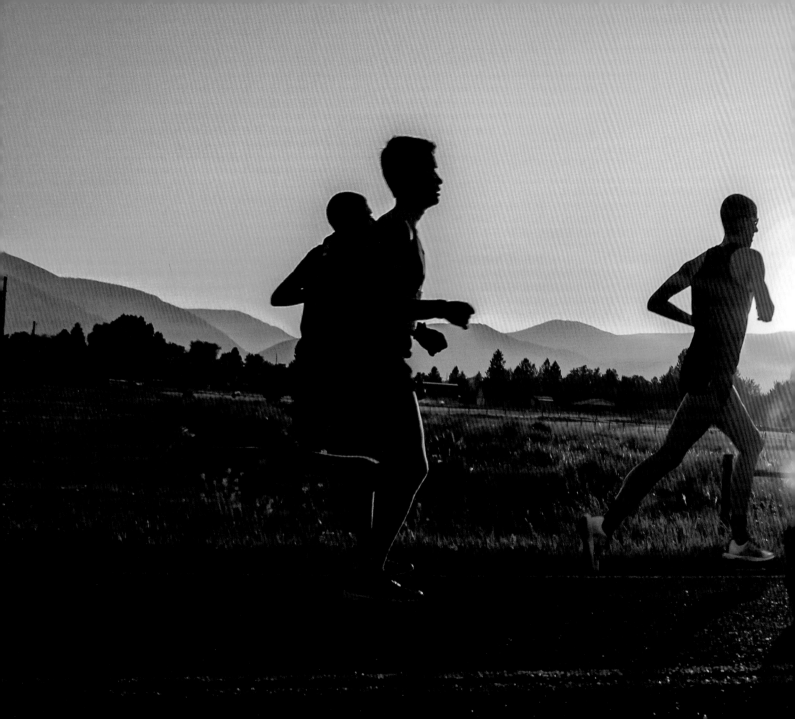

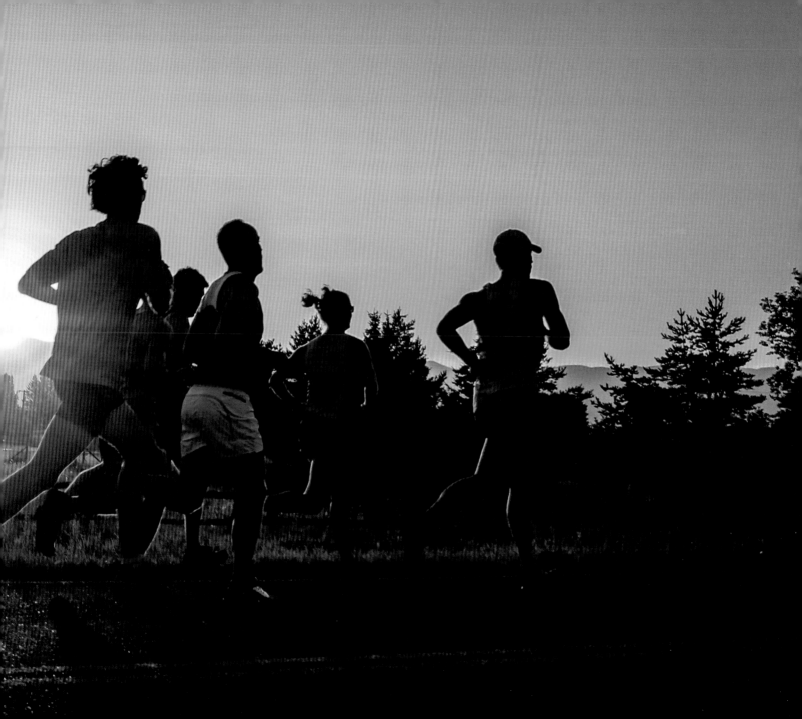

NUTRITION FACTS

BEFORE

	SERVES	CALORIES	PROTEIN	FAT	CARBS	FIBER	SODIUM
Apple Sandwiches	6	173	3	4	20	3.5	20
Apple Sweet Potato Mash	1	257	5	4	53	5	46
Beet Pistachio Bars	9	264	5	13	33	4	177
Beet Yogurt Bowl	6	237	10	4	42	4	250
Blender Beet Juice	2	119	3	1	29	1	126
Chocolate Banana Lettuce Wraps	1	203	3	7	35	4	34
Chocolate Quinoa Energy Balls	8	226	6	12	29	5	50
Coffee Concentrate (Cold-Brew Coffee) with ½ cup low-fat milk	6	52	4	1	6	0	56
Espresso Fruit Log	8	187	5.5	5	36	5	4
Graham Cracker Pumpkin Butter Smash	8	176	2.5	4	34	3	121
Instant Porridge	·	·	·	·	·	·	·
Apple Cinnamon	4	212	4	8	33	5	79
Apricot Ginger	4	221	6	8	35	5	77
Curry Cashew	4	249	6	10	38	4	81
Mocha	4	231	6	9	36	5	77
PB&J	4	174	7	3	32	5	148
Java Chia Pudding	2	260	6	13	36	11	76
Maple Millet Pudding	6	153	3	3	28	3	107

	SERVES	CALORIES	PROTEIN	FAT	CARBS	FIBER	SODIUM
				PER SERVING			
Maté Ginger Elixir	4	9	0	0	2	0	0
Muesli Squares	12	118	3	6	18	2	66
Open-Faced Rice Cake Sandwiches	.	.	.	.	.	.	.
Back in Black	4	98	6	2	16	2	30
Berry Hummus	4	109	3	3	8	3	143
Blueberry Cheesecake	4	194	6	12	17	2	89
Nutty Pear	4	115	4	3	19	3	82
Orange Crush Power Bites	8	150	2	11	14	3	56
Pumpkin Date Muffins	12	214	4	12	26	5	57
Raspberry Chia Pudding	2	200	5	9	28	13	140
Rice con Leche	1	269	6	8	48.5	3	11
Stuffed Dates	.	.	.	.	.	.	.
Citrus Ricotta	8	154	3	1	37	3	20
Coconut Zing	8	208	2	7	38	5	4
Open Sesame	8	222	3	8	39	4	6
Watermelon Slushy	1	118	2	0.5	31	1	4

DURING

	SERVES	CALORIES	PROTEIN	FAT	CARBS	FIBER	SODIUM
				PER SERVING			
Apricot Banana Sammies	8	82	1	2	17	2	27
Blini Sliders	.	.	.	.	.	.	.
Apple Pork	12	96	5	3	12	0	158
Cherry Cheesecake	12	106	3	3	16	1	57
Coco Choco	12	144	3.5	9	12	2	22
Brownie Bites	10	130	3	6	19	3	77
Carrot Cake Cookies	7	219	4	5.5	40	2	103

	SERVES	CALORIES	PROTEIN	FAT	CARBS	FIBER	SODIUM
				PER SERVING			
Coconut Rice Cakes	12	161	3	3	31	2	144
Crepe Rolls	·	·	·	·	·	·	·
Chocolaty Banana	8	261	7	14	28	2	106
Hawaiian Pizza	8	206	13	8	20	1	489
Pad Thai	8	233	9	11.5	24	1.5	259
Enduro Balls	18	177	4.5	9	22.5	3	35
Energy Shots	·	·	·	·	·	·	·
Berry Maple	2	136	0	0	34	1	188
Honey of an Apricot	2	95	1	0	25	0	148
PB&J	2	148	2	4	26	1.5	147
Perky Raisin	2	108	1	0	28	1	51
Fig Crumble Bars	12	292	4	10	48	4	63
Granola Bites	12	243	8	12	32	3	106
Hand Pies	·	·	·	·	·	·	·
Caprese	8	211	6	12	19	0	170
Nutty Mango	8	260	4	16	27	0	262
Savory Apple Pie	8	201	6	10	21	1	181
Hash Brown Bacon Patties	8	158	10	5	18	2	457
Inside-Out Pancakes	5	155	5.5	2	22	2	121
Mango Lime Bars	12	190	4	3	26	9.5	35
Maple Applesauce Rolls	5	358	7	5	73	5	453
Maple Banana Chips	4	79	1	0	20	2	74
Mediterranean Mini-Muffins	12	121	4.5	9	21	1	222
Millet Cherry Bars	9	229	4	12	28	3	131
Peanut Pretzel Squares	12	213	6	12	25	2	53

	SERVES	CALORIES	PROTEIN	FAT	CARBS	FIBER	SODIUM
				PER SERVING			
Pesto Potato Patties	5	154	4	8	17	2	114
Plantain Rice Wraps	6	370	8	7	69	5	567
Smoky Honey Mustard Bars	9	199	8	11	22	2	136
Sports Drinks	·	·	·	·	·	·	·
Ciderade	1	150	0	0	39	0	467
Maple Orange	1	214	2	0	52	0	442
Minty Pomegranate	1	140	0	0	35	0	459
Strawberry Cheesecake Wraps	6	308	8	12	43	4	355
Sweet Potato Tots	12	112	2	6	16	4	64
Sushi Rolls	5	314	15	3	53	1	811
Trail Mix	·	·	·	·	·	·	·
Cherry Haze	8	291	4	18	31	4	2
Crunchy Apple	8	213	5	16	25	5	7
Gourmet Pizza	8	191	7	12	16	3	312
Tropical Twister	8	214	6	10	27	4	62
Waffle Bites	·	·	·	·	·	·	·
Berry Chocolate	8	158	4	5	25	3	99
Waffle 'Zas	8	179	8	10	15	1	213
Zucchini Bread Bites	12	125	3	4	20	1	106

AFTER

	SERVES	CALORIES	PROTEIN	FAT	CARBS	FIBER	SODIUM
				PER SERVING			
Apricot Gazpacho	4	248	9	16	19	6	157
Apricot Grilled Cheese	6	288	14	10	37	6	454
Beast Bars	9	149	10	7	13	2	380
Blueberry Protein Freezer Pancakes	7	192	11	2	32	4	161
Cantaloupe Bowls with Crunchy Quinoa	2	256	14	4	47	4	48

AFTER *(contined)*

	SERVES	CALORIES	PROTEIN	FAT	CARBS	FIBER	SODIUM
Cereal and Milk	6	411	12	20	52	8	73
Cherry Mojito Popsicles	6	85	5	1	15	1	5
Chinese Pickled Eggs	4	97	7	5	5	0	595
Chocolate Avocado Pudding	4	325	13	16	41	11	92
Chocolate Milk	4	138	10	3	35	2	259
Edamame Hummus Wraps	6	376	14	20	37	6	707
Farro Egg Cakes	6	181	12	7	16	3	359
Flourless Protein Banana Muffins	12	183	8	10	18	2	69
Fruit and Grain Drink	4	166	3	0.5	41	3	5
Granola Pie	8	313	11	15	36	4	94
Granola Yogurt Bark	6	161	8	2	28	1	36
Hot Chocolate Recovery Smoothie	1	369	32	7	45	5	168
Instant Miso Noodle Soup	1	317	12	13	39	4	1,218
Molten Chocolate Mug Cake	1	312	22	13	30	3	249
Muesli Salad	4	540	30	31	38	6	204
PB&Berry Protein Oats	1	436	30	15	47	11	78
Pizza Mug Cake	1	405	15	25	30	1	389
Potato Pancake Smoked Fish Sandwiches	8	164	8	7	19	2	355
Pumpkin Pie Yogurt Bowl with Super Seed Sprinkle	4	307	1	16	30	3.5	31
Recovery Ice Cream	·	·	·	·	·	·	·
Gotcha Matcha	1	243	20	0	42	4	2
Mint Chip	1	441	14	17	59	8	6
PB&J	1	314	24	9	39	6	5
Peach Cheesecake	1	371	13	15	54	6	228
Salmon Salad Jars	2	551	34	24	54	8	442
Salmon Jerky	8	184	18	11	2		301
Salted Quinoa Almond Fudge Cups	12	177	7	13	13	1	3

	SERVES	PER SERVING					
		CALORIES	PROTEIN	FAT	CARBS	FIBER	SODIUM
Smoothie Cups	·	·	·	·	·	·	·
Cherry Cheesecake with 1 cup almond milk	6	194	14	11	19	3	361
Green Monster with 1 cup low-fat milk	6	292	16	12	34	6	162
Mocha Madness with 1 cup low-fat milk	6	283	17	12	31	5	131
Thai Mango Tango with 1 cup coconut milk bev.	6	194	7	11	22	2	26
Smoothie Packs	·	·	·	·	·	·	·
Green Power	4	377	14	16	50	16	523
Orange Crush	4	315	24	7	41	9	404
Spaghetti Bolognese Muffins	12	212	16	8	18	1	278
Sweet Potato Shake	1	426	16	9	75	7	173
Toast Stacks	·	·	·	·	·	·	·
Bean Good	4	266	10	12	33	9	559
Cottage Country	4	183	13	7	19	5	337
Go Fish	4	257	13	10	18	3	579
Going Bananas	4	295	27	11	23	6	274
Just Peachy	4	240	11	11	26	5	318
Turmeric Ginger Tonic	4	33	0	0	9	0	1
Tuna Balls	8	118	11	3	1	1	291
Turkey Muffins	12	192	15	9	12	2	158
Umami Tomato Juice	4	64	3	1	12	3	421

RESOURCES

Abeego
Earth-friendly, reusable, malleable food wraps. **www.abeego.com**

Ball
Iconic jars for packing your fuel, smoothies, and summer cocktails. **www.freshpreserving.com**

Bob's Red Mill
A bounty of fuel essentials such as flours and grains. **www.bobsredmill.com**

Cuisinart
Top-quality food processors and other useful kitchen gizmos. **www.cuisinart.com**

Eden Foods
Organic items packed in BPA-free cans. **www.edenfoods.com**

Hydro Flask
Top-notch insulated stainless-steel containers for food and beverages. **www.hydroflask.com**

Fridge-to-Go Cooler
Collapsible cooler that maintains refrigerator temperature for up to 12 hours, without electricity or ice packs. **www.fridge-to-go.com**

Justin's
Delicious nut butters and chocolate spreads. **www.justins.com**

Lodge
A stellar selection of pre-seasoned cast-iron cookware. **www.lodgemfg.com**

Madecasse
Chocolate and vanilla, the good stuff. **www.madecasse.com**

Made in Nature
Single-ingredient organic dried fruits. **www.madeinnature.com**

Manitoba Harvest
Top-notch hemp foods. **www.manitobaharvest.com**

Mastrad
Kitchen gizmos like scales, silicon baking pans, and oil misters. **www.mastrad-paris.us**

Microplane
High-quality zesters. **www.microplane.com**

Navitas Naturals
A broad range of superfoods, including raw cacao powder, cacao nibs, and chia seeds. **www.navitasnaturals.com**

Nutiva
All things hemp, chia, and coconut, including coconut butter and flour. **www.nutiva.com**

PaperChef
Parchment paper and nonstick muffin cup liners. **www.paperchef.com**

Trudeau
Silicone-based baking pans. **www.trudeaucorp.com**

Wild Planet
Sustainably caught canned seafood packed in BPA-free tins. **www.wildplanetfoods.com**

BIBLIOGRAPHY

Introduction

An, R. 2015. "Fast-Food and Full-Service Restaurant Consumption and Daily Energy and Nutrient Intakes in US Adults." *European Journal of Clinical Nutrition* July 1. doi:10.1038/ejcn.2015.104.

An, R., et al. 2015. "Fast-Food and Full-Service Restaurant Consumption in Relation to Daily Energy and Nutrient Intakes Among US Adult Cancer Survivors, 2003–2012." *Nutrition and Health* Aug. 6. doi: 10.1177/0260106015594098.

Zaupa, M., et al. 2015. "Characterization of Total Antioxidant Capacity and (Poly)phenolic Compounds of Differently Pigmented Rice Varieties and Their Changes During Domestic Cooking." *Food Chemistry* 187:338–47.

Before

Alkhatib, A. 2014. "Yerba Maté (*Illex paraguariensis*) Ingestion Augments Fat Oxidation and Energy Expenditure During Exercise at Various Submaximal Intensities." *Nutrition and Metabolism* 11:42.

Berry, M. J., et al. 2015. "Dietary Nitrate Supplementation Improves Exercise Performance and Decreases Blood Pressure in COPD Patients." *Nitric Oxide* 48:22–30.

Davison, G., et al. 2012. "The Effect of Acute Pre-exercise Dark Chocolate Consumption on Plasma Antioxidant Status, Oxidative Stress and Immunoendocrine Responses to Prolonged Exercise." *European Journal of Nutrition* 51 (1): 69–79.

Dugas, J. 2011. "Ice Slurry Ingestion Increases Running Time in the Heat." *Clinical Journal of Sports Medicine* 21 (6): 541–2.

Haakonssen, E. C., et al. 2014. "Dairy-Based Preexercise Meal Does Not Affect Gut Comfort or Time-Trial Performance in Female Cyclists." *International Journal of Sports Nutrition and Exercise Metabolism* 24 (5): 553–8.

Hall, K. D., et al. 2015. "Calorie for Calorie, Dietary Fat Restriction Results in More Body Fat Loss Than Carbohydrate Restriction in People with Obesity." *Cell Metabolism* 22 (3): 427–36.

Hardy, K., et al. 2015. "The Importance of Dietary Carbohydrate in Human Evolution." *The Quarterly Review of Biology* 90 (3): 251–68.

Illian, T. G., et al. 2011. "Omega 3 Chia Seed Loading as a Means of Carbohydrate Loading." *Journal of Strength and Conditioning Research* 25 (1): 61–5.

Jaceldo-Siegl, K., et al. 2014. "Tree Nuts Are Inversely Associated with Metabolic Syndrome and Obesity: The Adventist Health Study-2." *PLoS One* 9 (1): e85133.

Jackson, C. L., et al. 2014. "Long-Term Associations of Nut Consumption with Body Weight and Obesity." *American Journal of Clinical Nutrition* 100 (Suppl. 1): 408S–11S.

Judelson, D. A., et al. 2008. "Effect of Hydration State on Resistance Exercise–Induced Endocrine Markers of Anabolism, Catabolism, and Metabolism." *Journal of Applied Physiology* 105 (3): 816–24.

Karamanolis, I. A., et al. 2011. "The Effects of Pre-exercise Glycemic Index Food on Running Capacity." *International Journal of Sports Medicine* 32 (9): 666–71.

Kirwan, J. P., et al. 2001. "Effects of Moderate and High Glycemic Index Meals on Metabolism and Exercise Performance." *Metabolism* 50 (7): 849–55.

Lee, J. S., et al. 2015. "Effects of Chronic Dietary Nitrate Supplementation on the Hemodynamic Response to Dynamic Exercise." *American Journal of Physiology—Regulatory, Integrative and Comparative Physiology* June 17. doi:10.1152/ajpregu.00099.2015.

Little, J. P., et al. 2010. "Effect of Low- and High-Glycemic-Index Meals on Metabolism and Performance During High-Intensity, Intermittent Exercise." *International Journal of Sports Nutrition and Exercise Metabolism* 20 (6): 447–56.

Mariotti Lippi, M., et al. 2015. "Multistep Food Plant Processing at Grotta Paglicci (Southern Italy) Around 32,600 Cal B.P." *Proceedings of the National Academy of Sciences of the United States of America* Sept. 8. doi:10.1073/pnas.1516217112.

Morris, N. B., et al. 2015. "Ice Slurry Ingestion Leads to a Lower Net Heat Loss During Exercise in the Heat." *Medicine and Science in Sports and Exercise* Aug. 7. doi:10.1249/MSS.0000000000000746.

Peeling, P., et al. 2015. "Beetroot Juice Improves On-Water 500 M Time-Trial Performance, and Laboratory-Based Paddling Economy in National and International-Level Kayak Athletes." *International Journal of Sports Nutrition and Exercise Metabolism* 25 (3): 278–84.

Tarazona-Díaz, M. P., et al. 2013. "Watermelon Juice: Potential Functional Drink for Sore Muscle Relief in Athletes." *Journal of Agricultural and Food Chemistry* 61 (31): 7522–8.

During

Baker, L. B., et al. 2015. "Acute Effects of Carbohydrate Supplementation on Intermittent Sports Performance." *Nutrients* 7 (7): 5733–63.

Benton, D., et al. 2015. "Executive Summary and Conclusions from the European Hydration Institute Expert Conference on Human Hydration, Health, and Performance." *Nutrition Reviews* 73 (Suppl. 2): 148–50.

Brukner, P. 2013. "Challenging Beliefs in Sports Nutrition: Are Two 'Core Principles' Proving to Be Myths Ripe for Busting?" *British Journal of Sports Medicine* 47 (11): 663–4.

Burdon, C., et al. 2010. "Effect of Drink Temperature on Core Temperature and Endurance Cycling Performance in Warm, Humid Conditions." *Journal of Sports Sciences* 28 (11): 1147–56.

Burdon, C. A., et al. 2010. "Influence of Beverage Temperature on Exercise Performance in the Heat: A Systematic Review." *International Journal of Sports Nutrition and Exercise Science* 20 (2): 166–74.

Carter, J. M., et al. 2004. "The Effect of Carbohydrate Mouth Rinse on 1-H Cycle Time Trial Performance." *Medicine and Science in Sports and Exercise* 36 (12): 2107–11.

Casa, D. J., et al. 2000. "National Athletic Trainers' Association Position Statement: Fluid Replacement for Athletes." *Journal of Athletic Training* 35 (2): 212–24.

Cermak, N. M. and van Loon, L. J. 2013. "The Use of Carbohydrates During Exercise as an Ergogenic Aid." *Sports Medicine* 43 (11): 1139–55.

Cochran, A. J., et al. 2015. "Manipulating Carbohydrate Availability Between Twice-Daily Sessions of High-Intensity Interval Training over Two Weeks Improves Time-Trial Performance." *International Journal of Sports Nutrition and Exercise Metabolism* March 26.

Coombes, J. S., et al. 2000. "The Effectiveness of Commercially Available Sports Drinks." *Sports Medicine* 29 (3): 181–209.

Coyle, E. F., et al. 1986. "Muscle Glycogen Utilization During Prolonged Strenuous Exercise When Fed Carbohydrate." *Journal of Applied Physiology* 61 (1): 165–72.

Del Coso, J., et al. 2015. "Effects of Oral Salt Supplementation on Physical Performance During a Half-Ironman: A Randomized Controlled Trial." *Scandinavian Journal of Medicine and Science in Sports* Feb. 14. doi:10.111/sms.12427.

Earnest, C. P., et al. 2004. "Low vs. High Glycemic Index Carbohydrate Gel Ingestion During Simulated 64-km Cycling Time Trial Performance." *Journal of Strength and Conditioning Research* 18 (3): 466–72.

Godek, S. F., et al. 2010. "Sweat Rates, Sweat Sodium Concentrations, and Sodium Losses in 3 Groups of Professional Football Players." *Journal of Athletic Training* 45 (4): 364–71

Harper, L. D., et al. 2015. "Physiological and Performance Effects of Carbohydrate Gels Consumed Prior to the Extra-Time Period of Prolonged Simulated Soccer Match-Play." *Journal of Science and Medicine in Sport* (June).

Jeukendrup, A. 2007. "Carbohydrate Supplementation During Exercise: Does It Help? How Much Is Too Much?" *Sports Science Exchange* 20 (3): 1–8. http://www.gssiweb.org/Article/sse-106-carbohydrate-supplementation-during-exercise-does-it-help-how-much-is-too-much-.

Jeukendrup, A. E., et al. 2010. "Carbohydrate and Exercise Performance: The Role of Multiple Transportable Carbohydrates." *Current Opinion in Clinical Nutrition and Metabolic Care* 13 (4): 452–7.

Lafata, D., et al. 2012. "The Effect of a Cold Beverage During an Exercise Session Combining Both Strength and Energy Systems Development Training on Core Temperature and Markers of Performance." *Journal of the International Society of Sports Nutrition* 9 (1): 44.

Lane, S. C., et al. 2013. "Effect of a Carbohydrate Mouth Rinse on Simulated Cycling Time-Trial Performance Commenced in a Fed or Fasted State." *American Physiology, Nutrition, and Metabolism* 38 (2): 134–9.

Maughan, R. J., et al. 2004. "Fluid and Electrolyte Intake and Loss in Elite Soccer Players During Training." *International Journal of Sports Nutrition and Exercise Metabolism* 14 (3): 333–46.

Maughan, R. J., et al. 2015. "Implications of Active Lifestyles and Environmental Factors for Water Needs and Consequences of Failure to Meet Those Needs." *Nutrition Reviews* 73 (Suppl. 2): 130–40.

McGawley, K., et al. 2012. "Ingesting a High-Dose Carbohydrate Solution During the Cycle Section of a Simulated Olympic-Distance Triathlon Improves Subsequent Run Performance." *Applied Physiology, Nutrition, and Metabolism* 37 (4): 664–71.

McLellan, T. M., et al. 2014. "Effects of Protein in Combination with Carbohydrate Supplements on Acute or Repeat Endurance Exercise Performance: A Systematic Review." *Sports Medicine* 44 (4): 535–50.

Morris, J. G., et al. 2003. "The Influence of a 6.5% Carbohydrate-Electrolyte Solution on Performance of Prolonged Intermittent High-Intensity Running at 30 Degrees C." *Journal of Sport Sciences* 21 (5): 371–81.

Mündel, T., et al. 2006. "Drink Temperature Influences Fluid Intake and Endurance Capacity in Men During Exercise in a Hot, Dry Environment." *Experimental Physiology* 91 (5): 925–33.

Murray, R., et al. 1999. "A Comparison of the Gastric Emptying Characteristics of Selected Sports Drinks." *International Journal of Sports Nutrition* 9 (3): 263–74.

Newell, M. L., et al. 2015. "The Ingestion of 39 or 64 g·h-1 of Carbohydrate Is Equally Effective at Improving Endurance Exercise Performance in Cyclists." *International Journal of Sports Nutrition and Exercise Metabolism* 25 (3): 285–92.

Nieman, D. C., et al. 2012. "Bananas as an Energy Source During Exercise: A Metabolomics Approach." *PLoS One* 7 (5): e37479.

Oosthuyse, T., et al. 2015. "Whey or Casein Hydrolysate with Carbohydrate for Metabolism and Performance in Cycling." *International Journal of Sports Medicine* 36 (8): 636–46.

Phillips, S. M., et al. 2011. "Carbohydrate Ingestion During Team Games Exercise: Current Knowledge and Areas for Future Investigation." *Sports Medicine* 41 (7): 559–85.

Rontoyanni, V. G., et al. 2015. "Differential Acute Effects of Carbohydrate- and Protein-Rich Drinks Compared with Water on Cardiac Output During Rest and Exercise in Healthy Young Men." *Applied Physiology, Nutrition, and Metabolism* 40 (8): 803–10.

Rowlands, D. S., et al. 2011. "Unilateral Fluid Absorption and Effects on Peak Power After Ingestion of Commercially Available Hypotonic, Isotonic, and Hypertonic Sports Drinks." *International Journal of Sports Nutrition and Metabolism* 21 (6): 480–91.

Saunders, M. J. 2007. "Coingestion of Carbohydrate-Protein During Endurance Exercise: Influence on Performance and Recovery." *International Journal of Sports Nutrition and Exercise Metabolism* 17 (Suppl.): S87–103.

Schlader, Z. J., et al. "Fluid Restriction During Exercise in the Heat Reduces Tolerance to Progressive Central Hypovolaemia." *Experimental Physiology* 100 (8): 926–34.

Sun, F. H., et al. "Carbohydrate Electrolyte Solutions Enhance Endurance Capacity in Active Females." *Nutrients* 7 (5): 3739–50.

Too, B. W., et al. 2012. "Natural Versus Commercial Carbohydrate Supplementation and Endurance Running Performance." *Journal of the International Society of Sports Nutrition* 9 (1): 27.

van Loon, L. J., et al. 2001. "The Effects of Increasing Exercise Intensity on Muscle Fuel Utilisation in Humans." *The Journal of Physiology* 536 (Pt 1): 295–304.

Welsh, R. S., et al. 2002. "Carbohydrates and Physical/Mental Performance During Intermittent Exercise to Fatigue." *Medicine and Science in Sports and Exercise* 34 (4): 723–31.

Wilson, P. B., et al. 2014. "Glucose-Fructose Likely Improves Gastrointestinal Comfort and Endurance Running Performance Relative to Glucose-Only." *Scandinavian Journal of Medicine and Science in Sports* Dec. 30. doi:10.1111/sms.12386.

Wilson, P. B., et al. 2015. "Saccharide Composition of Carbohydrates Consumed During an Ultra-Endurance Triathlon." *Journal of the American College of Nutrition* May 5:1–10.

Yeo, W. K., et al. 2011. "Fat Adaptation in Well-Trained Athletes: Effects on Cell Metabolism." *Applied Physiology, Nutrition, and Metabolism* 36 (1): 12–22.

After

Aargon, A. A., et al. 2013. "Nutrient Timing Revisited: Is There a Post-Exercise Anabolic Window?" *Journal of the International Society of Sports Nutrition and Metabolism* 10 (5). doi:10.1186/1550-2783-10-5.

Alghannam, A. F., et al. 2015. "Impact of Muscle Glycogen Availability on the Capacity for Repeated Exercise in Man." *Medicine and Science in Sports and Exercise* July 20.

Bell, P. G., et al. 2014. "Montmorency Cherries Reduce the Oxidative Stress and Inflammatory Responses to Repeated Days of High-Intensity Stochastic Cycling." *Nutrients* 6 (2): 829–43.

Berardi, J. M., et al. 2008. "Recovery from a Cycling Time Trial Is Enhanced with Carbohydrate-Protein Supplementation vs. Isoenergetic Carbohydrate Supplementation." *Journal of the International Society of Sports Nutrition* 5:24.

Bishop, P. A., et al. 2008. "Recovery from Training: A Brief Review." *Journal of Strength and Conditioning Research* 22 (3): 1015–24.

Black, C. D., et al. 2010. "Ginger (*Zingiber officinale*) Reduces Muscle Pain Caused by Eccentric Exercise." *Journal of Pain* 11 (9): 894–903.

Bukhari, S. S., et al. 2015. "Intake of Low-Dose Leucine-Rich Essential Amino Acids Stimulates Muscle Anabolism Equivalently to Bolus Whey Protein in Older Women at Rest and After Exercise." *American Journal of Physiology* 308 (12): E1056–65.

Connolly, D. A., et al. 2006. "Efficacy of a Tart Cherry Juice Blend in Preventing the Symptoms of Muscle Damage." *British Journal of Sports Medicine* 40 (8): 679–83.

Cramer, M. J., et al. 2015. "Post-exercise Glycogen Recovery and Exercise Performance Is Not Significantly Different Between Fast Food and Sport Supplements." *International Journal of Sports Nutrition and Exercise Metabolism* March 26. doi:10.1123/ijsnem.2014-0230.

Desbrow, B., et al. 2014. "Comparing the Rehydration Potential of Different Milk-Based Drinks to a Carbohydrate-Electrolyte Beverage." *American Physiology, Nutrition, and Metabolism* 39 (12): 1366–72.

Devries, M. C., et al. 2015. "Supplemental Protein in Support of Muscle Mass and Health: Advantage Whey." *Journal of Food Science* 80 (Suppl. 1): A8–15.

Dimitriou, L., et al. 2015. "Influence of a Montmorency Cherry Juice Blend on Indices of Exercise-Induced Stress and Upper Respiratory Tract Symptoms Following Marathon Running—A Pilot Investigation." *Journal of the International Society of Sports Nutrition* 12:22.

Gil, J. H., et al. 2015. "Effects of Different Doses of Leucine Ingestion Following Eight Weeks of Resistance Exercise on Protein Synthesis and Hypertrophy of Skeletal Muscle in Rats." *Journal of Exercise Nutrition and Metabolism* 19 (1): 31–8.

Harms-Ringdahl, M., et al. 2012. "Tomato Juice Intake Suppressed Serum Concentration of 8-oxodG After Extensive Physical Activity." *Nutrition Journal* 11:29.

Haywood, B. A., et al. 2014. "Probiotic Supplementation Reduces the Duration and Incidence of Infections but Not Severity in Elite Rugby Union Players." *Journal of Science in Sports and Medicine* 17 (4): 356–60.

Hill, A. M., et al. 2007. "Combining Fish-Oil Supplements with Regular Aerobic Exercise Improves Body Composition and Cardiovascular Disease Risk Factors." *American Journal of Clinical Nutrition* 85 (5): 1267–74.

Ivy, J. L. 1998. "Glycogen Resynthesis After Exercise: Effect of Carbohydrate Intake." *International Journal of Sports Medicine* 19 (Suppl. 2): S142–5.

Ivy, J. L., et al. 2004. "Regulation of Muscle Glycogen Repletion, Muscle Protein Synthesis and Repair Following Exercise." *Journal of Sports Science and Medicine* 3:131–38.

Jentjens, R., et al. 2003. "Determinants of Post-exercise Glycogen Synthesis During Short-Term Recovery." *Sports Medicine* 33 (2): 117–44.

Kato, H., et al. 2015. "Leucine-Enriched Essential Amino Acids Attenuate Muscle Soreness and Improve Muscle Protein Synthesis After Eccentric Contractions in Rats." *Amino Acids* 47 (6): 1193–201.

Layman, D. K., et al. 2009. "Egg Protein as a Source of Power, Strength and Energy." *Nutrition Today* 44 (1): 43–8.

Lembke, et al. 2014. "Influence of Omega-3 (N3) Index on Performance and Wellbeing in Young Adults After Heavy Eccentric Exercise." *Journal of Sports Science and Medicine* 13 (1): 151–6.

Lis, D., et al. 2015. "No Effects of a Short-Term Gluten-Free Diet on Performance in Nonceliac Athletes." *Medicine and Science in Sports and Exercise.* 47(12):2563–70.

Lowery, L. M. and Antonio, J. 2012. *Dietary Protein and Resistance Exercise*. Boca Raton: FL: CRC Press.

Lunn, W. R., et al. 2012. "Chocolate Milk and Endurance Exercise Recovery: Protein Balance, Glycogen, and Performance." *Medicine and Science in Sports and Exercise* 44 (4): 682–91.

Melzer, D., et al. 2012. "Urinary Bisphenol A Concentration and Risk of Future Coronary Artery Disease in Apparently Healthy Men and Women." *Circulation* 125 (12): 1482–90.

Moore, D. R., et al. 2009. "Ingested Protein Dose Response of Muscle and Albumin Protein Synthesis After Resistance Exercise in Young Men." *American Journal of Clinical Nutrition* 89 (1): 161–8.

Moore, D. R., et al. 2015. "Nutrition to Support Recovery from Endurance Exercise: Optimal Carbohydrate and Protein Replacement." *Current Sports Medicine Reports* 14 (4): 294–300.

Nicol, L. M., et al. 2015. "Curcumin Supplementation Likely Attenuates Delayed Onset Muscle Soreness (DOMS)." *European Journal of Applied Physiology* 115 (8): 1769–77.

Outlaw, J. J., et al. 2014. "Effects of a Pre- and Post-workout Protein-Carbohydrate Supplement in Trained Crossfit Individuals." *SpringerPlus* 3:369.

Pasiakos, S. M., et al. 2015. "The Effects of Protein Supplements on Muscle Mass, Strength, and Aerobic and Anaerobic Power in Healthy Adults: A Systematic Review." *Sports Medicine* 45 (1): 111–31.

Pritchett, K., et al. 2009. "Acute Effects of Chocolate Milk and a Commercial Recovery Beverage on Postexercise Recovery Indices and Endurance Cycling Performance." *Applied Physiology, Nutrition, and Metabolism* 34 (6): 1017–22.

Song, Y., et al. 2014. "Urinary Concentrations of Bisphenol A and Phthalate Metabolites and Weight Change: A Prospective Investigation in US Women." *International Journal of Obesity* 38 (12): 1532–7.

Spaccarotella, K. J., et al. 2011. "The Effects of Low Fat Chocolate Milk on Postexercise Recovery in Collegiate Athletes." *The Journal of Strength and Conditioning Research* 25 (12): 3456–60.

van Vliet, S., et al. 2015. "The Skeletal Muscle Anabolic Response to Plant- Versus Animal-Based Protein Consumption." *The Journal of Nutrition* 145 (9): 1981–91.

Volterman, K. A., et al. 2014. "Effect of Milk Consumption on Rehydration in Youth Following Exercise in the Heat." *Applied Physiology, Nutrition, and Metabolism* 39 (11): 1257–64.

Volterman, K. A., et al. 2014. "Effects of Postexercise Milk Consumption on Whole Body Protein Balance in Youth." *Journal of Applied Physiology* 117 (10): 1165–9.

Żebrowska, A., et al. 2015. "Omega-3 Fatty Acids Supplementation Improves Endothelial Function and Maximal Oxygen Uptake in Endurance-Trained Athletes." *European Journal of Sports Science* 15 (4): 305–14.

INDEX

ABOUT THE AUTHOR

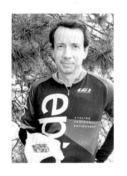

Matthew Kadey is a registered dietitian, freelance nutrition writer, and recipe developer based in Waterloo, Ontario, Canada. As a prolific magazine writer, his nutrition, recipe, and travel articles have appeared in dozens of publications including *Bicycling*, *Runner's World*, *Men's Health*, *Vegetarian Times*, *Triathlete*, *Women's Health*, *Muscle & Fitness*, *Shape*, *Eating Well*, and *Men's Fitness*. He received a master's degree in sports nutrition from Florida State University and a prestigious 2013 James Beard Award for food journalism. He is also the author of *Muffin Tin Chef: 101 Savory Snacks, Adorable Appetizers, Enticing Entrees and Delicious Desserts*, and *The No-Cook, No-Bake Cookbook*. As an avid two-wheeled tourist, Matt has cycled and feasted his way through numerous countries including Chile, Mexico, New Zealand, Myanmar, Sri Lanka, Laos, Thailand, Cuba, Ireland, Ethiopia, Belize, and Jordan. He is also a former provincial mountain bike champion in his age category. You can find Matt at www.mattkadey.com or at www.rocketfuelfoods.net.

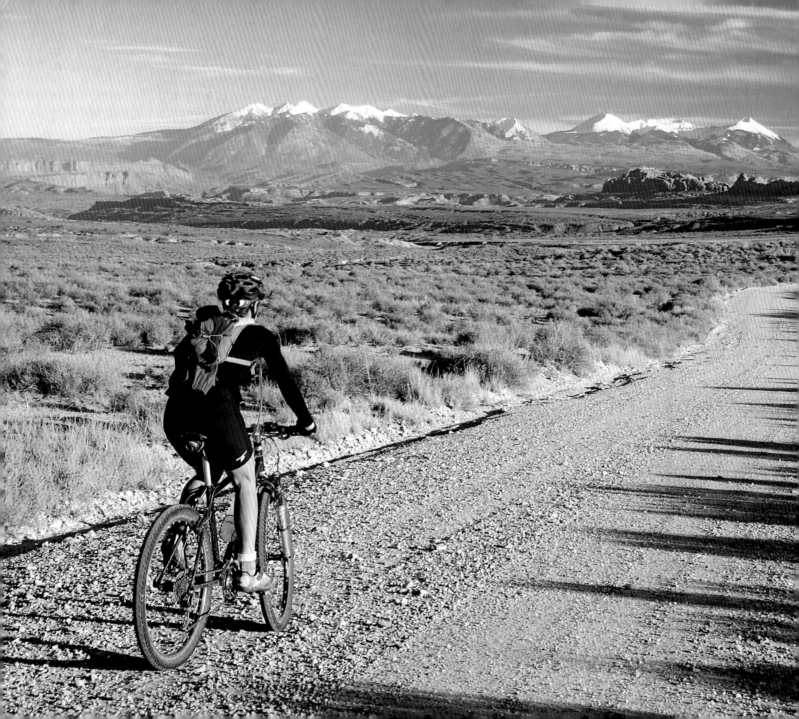